Pain Management

Editor

LYNN C. PARSONS

CRITICAL CARE NURSING CLINICS OF NORTH AMERICA

www.ccnursing.theclinics.com

December 2024 • Volume 36 • Number 4

ELSEVIER

1600 John F. Kennedy Boulevard • Suite 1800 • Philadelphia, Pennsylvania, 19103-2899

http://www.theclinics.com

CRITICAL CARE NURSING CLINICS OF NORTH AMERICA Volume 36, Number 4
December 2024 ISSN 0899-5885, ISBN-13: 978-0-443-29352-8

Editor: Kerry Holland
Developmental Editor: Sukirti Singh

Critical Care Nursing Clinics of North America (ISSN 0899-5885) is published quarterly by Elsevier Inc., 360 Park Avenue South, New York, NY 10010-1710. Months of issue are March, June, September, and December. Business and Editorial Offices: 1600 John F. Kennedy Blvd., Suite 1800, Philadelphia, PA 19103-2899. Periodicals postage paid at New York, NY and additional mailing offices. Subscription prices are $166.00 per year for US individuals, $100.00 per year for US students and residents, $206.00 per year for Canadian individuals, $230.00 per year for international individuals, $115.00 per year for international students/residents and $100.00 per year for Canadian students/residents. For institutional access pricing please contact Customer Service via the contact information below. To receive student/resident rate, orders must be accompanied by name of affiliated institution, data of term, and the *signature* of program/residency coordinator on institution letterhead. Orders will be billed at individual rate until proof of status is received. Foreign air speed delivery is included in all *Clinics* subscription prices. All prices are subject to change without notice. Orders, claims, and journal inquiries: Please visit our Support Hub page https://service.elsevier.com for assistance.

Reprints. For copies of 100 or more of articles in this publication, please contact the Commercial Reprints Department, Elsevier Inc., 360 Park Avenue South, New York, New York, 10010-1710; Tel.: 212-633-3874, Fax: 212-633-3820, and E-mail: reprints@elsevier.com.

Critical Care Nursing Clinics of North America is covered in *MEDLINE/PubMed (Index Medicus), International Nursing Index, Nursing Citation Index, Cumulative Index to Nursing and Allied Health Literature,* and *RNdex Top 100.*

Contributors

EDITOR

LYNN C. PARSONS, PhD, RN, NEA-BC
C. Louise Caudill Professor and Department Chair, Department of Nursing, School of Health Sciences, Morehead State University, Center for Health, Education and Research, Morehead, Kentucky

AUTHORS

MAHALIA G. BARROW, EdD, RN, CNL
Clinical Assistant Professor, Capstone College of Nursing, The University of Alabama in Tuscaloosa, Tuscaloosa, Alabama

AMI BHATT, PhD, DNP, MBA, RN
Core Faculty, College of Nursing, Walden University, Minneapolis, Minnesota

AVANI BHATT, MSN, RN
Critical Care Nurse, Trinity Health-Ann Arbor Hospital, Ypsilanti, Michigan

KRISTEN BUTLER, DNP, MSN, RN
Associate Professor of Nursing, Austin Peay State University, Clarksville, Tennessee

HEATHER S. COLE, PhD, RN, CHSE, CNEN
Assistant Professor, Director of Clinical Simulation, Capstone College of Nursing, The University of Alabama in Tuscaloosa, Tuscaloosa, Alabama

TERESA ELLETT, DNP, MSN, BSN, RN, CNE
Professor of Nursing, Morehead State University, Morehead, Kentucky

CHRISTINE FRAZER, PhD, CNS, CNE
Senior Core Faculty, College of Nursing, Walden University, Minneapolis, Minnesota

BENJAMIN A. FUJITA-HOWIE, MD, MPH
Resident Doctor, Pain Medicine Department, Icahn School of Medicine at Mount Sinai, New York, New York

WILLIAM O. HOWIE, CRNA, DNP, FAANA
Staff Nurse Anesthetist, R. Adams Cowley Shock Trauma Center, Millersville, Maryland

PATRICIA C. McMULLEN, PhD, JD, CRNP, FAANP, FAAN
Dean Emerita and Ordinary Professor, Conway School of Nursing, The Catholic University of America, Millersville, Maryland

PRESTON H. MILLER, PhD, RN, CCRN-CMC, PCCN, CFRN
Assistant Professor, Department of Nursing, University of Alabama in Huntsville College of Nursing, Huntsville, Alabama

HEATHER MORAN, MSN, RN, CRRN, CMSRN, CNE
Assistant Professor of Nursing, Austin Peay State University, Clarksville, Tennessee

JEANNE MORRISON, PhD, MSN
Nurse Executive Coordinator, College of Nursing, Walden University, Minneapolis, Minnesota

MARY MORRISON, BS
College of Psychology Doctoral Program, Walden University, Minneapolis, Minnesota

JENNY PAPPAS, DNP, APRN, FNP-C
Assistant Professor of Nursing, Austin Peay State University, Clarksville, Tennessee

LYNN C. PARSONS, PhD, RN, NEA-BC
C. Louise Caudill Professor and Department Chair, Department of Nursing, School of Health Sciences, Morehead State University, Center for Health, Education and Research, Morehead, Kentucky

SHANNON L. SMITH-STEPHENS, DNP, APRN-BC, SANE
Family Nurse Practitioner, Owner/Provider, SSS Medical, Inc., Olive Hill; Contract Medical Provider, Department of Juvenile Justice, Frankfort, Kentucky

DEBRA SULLIVAN, PhD, MSN, RN, CNE, COI
Senior Core Faculty, College of Nursing, Walden University, Minneapolis, Minnesota

LORI A. SUTTON, MSN, RN
Assistant Professor of Nursing, Austin Peay State University, Clarksville, Tennessee

MARY SUZANNE WHITE, DNP, RN, PHCNS-BC
Associate Professor of Nursing, School of Health Sciences, Morehead State University, Morehead, Kentucky

LISA WALLACE, DNP, MSN, RN, RNC-OB, NE-BC
Associate Professor of Nursing, Morehead State University, Morehead, Kentucky

DEBRA ROSE WILSON, PhD, MSN, RN, IBCLC, AHN-BC, CHT
Professor of Nursing, Austin Peay State University, Walden University, Clarksville, Tennessee

STEVEN WOODEN, DNP, CRNA, NSPM-C
Adjunct Faculty School of Nurse Anesthesia, Texas Christian University, Fort Worth, Texas

GEORGE A. ZANGARO, PhD, RN, FAAN
Chief Policy and Scientific Officer, American Association of Colleges of Nursing, Washington, DC

Contents

> Managing pain, whether acute or chronic, has taken a whole new look during the past 3 decades. Pain management continues to be a long-standing public health concern. The ongoing opioid epidemic has changed how the term pain is not only treated but viewed throughout all lenses of society. The following content will focus on pain management of clients aged 18 years or older with acute and/or chronic pain in the outpatient setting. As advocates and gatekeepers, primary care providers must have knowledge of evidence-based guidelines and recommendations of pain management to provide the competent, holistic care and education clients deserve.

> This article examines the pivotal role of critical care nurses in managing pediatric pain, emphasizing the multifaceted nature of care. It covers the challenges and opportunities nurses face, stressing the importance of education and training. The background section underscores the global issue of inadequately managed pediatric pain and the importance of addressing social determinants of health while recognizing perceptions, beliefs, stereotypes, and biases on pain management. A multimodal approach in treatment is detailed in pharmacologic and non-pharmacologic approaches. Barriers nurses encounter are discussed, with recommendations for a holistic and individualized approach to pediatric pain management in critical care settings.

> The study is a longitudinal review of pain management claims filed in the state of Maryland. Adverse outcomes associated with pain-related claims are often severe and include death, brain damage, and back and spinal cord sequelae. There is a lot to be learned from past experiences, identified in closed pain management claims, specifically on how to improve patient education, outcomes, quality, and safety.

> Around 51.6 million adults are living with chronic pain that has been linked to mental health disorders, substance use, and suicidal ideation. The high incidence of chronic pain poses a challenge for health care educators to ensure that health care professionals receive training to assess, prevent, and manage chronic pain for a diverse patient population. While simulation-based learning is known as an effective educational strategy, little is known about its use to illustrate pain. This review aims to determine the current evidence related to using simulation-based learning for training and teaching the assessment and management of pain in nursing.

> Circumcision is a painful procedure that may be performed on newborns. Pain management is provided through pharmacologic and nonpharmacological methods such as administration of anesthetics, analgesia, nutritive sucking, music, and touch during and post procedure. Pain scales may be used to assess physiologic and behavioral changes in the newborn as part of the pain management process. The role of the nurse includes assisting the provider with pain management, assessing newborn pain, and teaching the family how to care and comfort the newborn post circumcision.

> The primary objective of this article is to share effective strategies for integrating patients and their families into the critical care setting. Additionally, it aims to address lack of pain management knowledge, burnout syndrome, and stress management tactics tailored for practicing critical care registered nurses.

> For centuries, pharmacologic interventions have been the primary intervention for pain in intensive care patients. Opioid use has significant side effects and long-term risks including addiction and loss of life. Critical care nurses and other health care professionals can include effective nonpharmacological complementary modalities to reduce pain. Approaches discussed include guided imagery, acupuncture, music and sound therapy, cold therapy, massage, and physical and occupational therapy. Evidence-based research that examined the efficacy of these complementary methods found significant reduction in pain, trauma, length of stay, or post-intensive care syndrome in critical care patients.

> Pain experienced by mechanically ventilated patients in intensive care units (ICUs) is often overlooked, but it is a significant issue. With over 5 million

annual ICU admissions in the United States, the prevalence of pain during hospitalization and its aftermath is a pressing concern. Chronic pain in ICU survivors has been linked to post-traumatic stress disorder, poor quality of life, and long-term impairments known as postintensive care syndrome. Barriers to effective pain management include psychological factors, sedation restrictions, and inadequate use of valid assessment tools.

Nurses have an ethical responsibility to manage pain and the suffering derived from it. Given the complexity of patients in the critical care setting and the high incidence of pain experienced by critically ill patients, critical care nurses may experience moral distress when pain is inadequately managed. To address moral distress associated with pain management, critical care nurses should be provided with education on evidence-based pain management practices and encouraged to evaluate their personal biases and beliefs regarding pain management. Furthermore, organizations should consider the implementation of programs to address moral distress stemming from pain management and other precipitating factors.

Hip fractures in women are a serious health concern, demanding prompt treatment and pain control methods. This study examines fracture frequency, diagnostic techniques, and classification, focusing on femoral neck and intertrochanteric fractures. It discusses risk factors including age, gender, bone strength, and medication and their impact on fracture risk. Treatments range from noninvasive care to surgeries such as internal fixation and joint replacement. Perioperative measures such as anesthesia, antibiotics, and clot prevention to improve outcomes and lessen complications are also discussed. Postsurgery care emphasizes pain relief strategies, including opioids, nerve blocks, and modern methods such as real-time messaging for pain control.

Chronic pain is a devastating condition that impacts more than 50 million adults nationwide. It can lead to chronic opioid addiction, reduced quality of life, economic collapse, divorce, homelessness, and suicide. Chronic pain associated with surgical interventions is a common, but often misunderstood and misdiagnosed condition. Understanding chronic pain and the physical, psychological, and psychosocial links to chronic postsurgical pain can help nurses identify, prevent, or better treat the condition.

Palliative care has evolved from its religious and historical roots to a specialized medical discipline, emphasizing quality of life for patients with serious illnesses. The foundational work of pioneers in palliative care has shaped modern practices in symptom management, emotional support, and holistic care. Despite challenges in integrating palliative care in critical care settings and overcoming barriers such as limited provider availability, enhancing training and broadening the application of palliative principles remain essential. Palliative care is crucial, not just for end-of-life scenarios, but for managing severe illness at any stage, ensuring compassionate, patient-centered care.

Lynn C. Parsons

Nurses practicing in critical care units manage all forms of traumatic, acute, and chronic pain. Chronic pain must be managed in critical care scenarios to facilitate patient comfort and eventual recovery and healing. Patients with orthopedic injuries and conditions have distinct care needs that require specialized knowledge on the provider's part. Critical care nurses manage orthopedic traumatic injuries while simultaneously managing underlying acute orthopedic conditions. Pain experiences are individual to the person experiencing pain. The Internet is a rich source for pain-management materials that the critical care nurse should have in their resource repertoire.

CRITICAL CARE NURSING CLINICS OF NORTH AMERICA

SERIES OF RELATED INTEREST

Nursing Clinics of North America http://www.nursing.theclinics.com
Critical Care Clinics www.criticalcare.theclinics.com

THE CLINICS ARE AVAILABLE ONLINE!
Access your subscription at:
www.theclinics.com

Preface

Pain Management Across the Lifespan

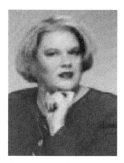

Lynn C. Parsons, PhD, RN, NEA-BC
Editor

In the health care landscape, nursing professionals shoulder the critical responsibility of managing patient pain. This is often the primary catalyst for individuals to seek medical care, underscoring the importance of its effective treatment.[1] Throughout their lives, patients grapple with both acute and chronic pain due to a range of afflictions, highlighting the need for nurses to have a thorough understanding of pain management.

The Cleveland Clinic[2] characterizes acute pain as a sudden discomfort triggered by a specific event or condition. This type of pain is typically associated with traumatic fractures, postoperative recovery, burns, abrasions, cuts, and active childbirth. It generally subsides once the underlying cause has been resolved and healed.

In contrast, chronic pain is a persistent discomfort that may last for more than 6 months.[2] It often continues even after the initial cause has healed and is commonly linked to conditions such as arthritis, back pain, and cancer.

Margo McCaffery, RN, MS, FAAN,[3] a trailblazing nurse leader in the field of pain interventions, has made significant strides in understanding and treating both acute and chronic pain across a variety of clinical settings throughout her distinguished career. Her 1968 definition of pain, "It's whatever the experiencing person says it is, existing whenever and wherever the person says it does," is widely embraced by today's clinicians.

In this issue, we delve into both acute and chronic pain conditions, including addiction, and explore treatment strategies for individuals across all life stages. We also discuss the importance of nurses being aware of social determinants of health when assessing pain. We scrutinize the latest evidence for pain management and a broad spectrum of treatment interventions implemented by nurses.

Crit Care Nurs Clin N Am 36 (2024) xi–xii
https://doi.org/10.1016/j.cnc.2024.04.002
0899-5885/24/© 2024 Published by Elsevier Inc.

ccnursing.theclinics.com

Our aim, through the provision of acute and chronic pain management strategies in this issue of *Critical Care Nursing Clinics of North America*, is to compile a comprehensive repository of pain management resources. These resources are designed to serve as practical tools for nurses on the frontlines of clinical practice, thereby benefiting our valued readership.

Lynn C. Parsons, PhD, RN, NEA-BC
School of Health Sciences
Morehead State University
Center for Health, Education and Research
316 West Second Street, CHER 201P
Morehead, KY 40351, USA

E-mail address:
Lynn.Parsons@mail.waldenu.edu

REFERENCES

1. Morton P, Thurman P. Critical care nursing: a holistic approach. 12th edition. The Netherlands: Wolters Kluwer; 2024.
2. Cleveland Clinic. Acute vs. chronic pain. 2020. Available at: https://my.cleveland clinic.org/health/articles/12051-acute-vs-chronic-pain. [Accessed 4 January 2024].
3. Pirschel C. Remembering Margo McCaffery's contributions to pain management. 2018. Available at: https://voice.ons.org/news-and-views/remembering-margo-mccafferys-contributions-to-pain-management. [Accessed 4 January 2024].

Managing Pain in an Era of Opioid Addiction

Shannon L. Smith-Stephens, DNP, APRN-BC, SANE[a,b,*]

KEYWORDS

- Pain • Acute pain • Chronic pain • Pain management • Substance abuse • Opioid

KEY POINTS

- Examine the definitions and diagnostic criteria of pain.
- Appraise the background and burden of disease related to the management of pain.
- Review guidelines and recommendations for therapeutic pain management of clients aged 18 years or older with acute and/or chronic pain in the outpatient setting with the exception of pain associated with cancer, sickle cell disease, or those receiving palliative or end-of-life care.

INTRODUCTION

Managing pain, whether acute or chronic, has taken a whole new appearance during the past 3 decades. Throughout history, one of the greatest medical challenges involves the conundrum of treating pain. Pain management has and continues to be a long-standing public health concern. The ongoing opioid epidemic has changed the scope of how the term pain is not only treated but also viewed throughout all lenses of society. This article will focus on pain management of clients aged 18 years or older with acute and/or chronic pain in the outpatient setting. The population of clients with pain associated with cancer, sickle cell disease, or those receiving palliative or end-of-life care is beyond the scope of this discussion.

BACKGROUND

Prescription opioid misuse and overdose deaths is at epidemic levels in the United States.

Schalkoff and colleagues[1] discussed the dramatic increase in overdose and overdose deaths seen in the United States during the last 30 to 40 years. At-risk populations and geographic locations have also shifted from African Americans in urban populations to young, White men in rural Appalachia. Young, White men in rural Appalachia with low levels of education, employment, and mental health disorders are among those at highest risk for substance use and overdose.[1] Buer, a public health

[a] SSS Medical, Inc., Olive Hill, KY, USA; [b] Department of Juvenile Justice
* 6902B Grahn Road, Olive Hill, KY 41164.
E-mail address: shannonsmithstephens@gmail.com

Crit Care Nurs Clin N Am 36 (2024) 469–477
https://doi.org/10.1016/j.cnc.2024.04.006

practitioner, looked at individualized stories of treatment and survival in Rural Kentucky, providing a gripping account of the substance abuse epidemic in Central Appalachia.[2] Buer also addressed the attention of undertreated pain in the early 1980s from the scope of patients, clinicians, and researchers, as well as recommendations from the American Pain Society.[2] Our society perceived pain was being undertreated, especially that of nonmalignant chronic pain. Prescription opioids were identified as beneficial for all patients, regardless of the likelihood of abuse or pain intensity. With the endorsement of prescription opioids, many health insurance companies suspended or limited funding of more holistic pain modalities such as occupational and psychological therapy, increasingly covering opioids as opposed to nonopioid treatment options. Thus, there are fewer options for chronic pain treatment in resource-poor areas, like Central Appalachia.[2] Review of the literature reveals consistent concerns regarding the lack of therapeutic options for pain management. A host of explanations ranging from inadequate clinician training and guidance, lack of pain management specialists, insufficient access to care, insurance coverage and reimbursement, implicit bias, and lack of supporting evidence for nonpharmacological pain modalities are a few of the rationales that have led to prescription opioids remaining as a cornerstone to treat pain.[3]

DIAGNOSTIC CRITERIA

In 2020, the International Association for the Study of Pain revised the definition of pain for the first time in over 40 years. Pain was defined as an unpleasant sensory and emotional experience associated with or resembling that associated with, actual or potential tissue damage, and is experienced upon by the addition of 6 key notes and the etymology of the word pain for further valuable content[4]:

- Pain is always a personal experience influenced by biological, psychological, and social factors.
- Pain and nociception are different phenomena. Pain cannot be inferred solely from activity in sensory neurons.
- Through their life experiences, individuals learn the concept of pain.
- A person's report of an experience of pain should be respected.
- Although pain usually serves an adaptive role, it may have adverse effects on function and social and psychological well-being.
- Verbal description is only one of several behaviors to express pain; inability to communicate does not negate the possibility that a human or a nonhuman animal experiences pain.

Pain is usually classified as acute (duration less than 1 month), subacute (duration of 1–3 months), and chronic (duration of >3 months). The American Academy of Pain Medicine defines acute pain as "the physiologic response and experience to noxious stimuli that can become pathologic, is normally sudden in onset, time limited, and motivates behaviors to avoid actual or potential tissue injuries."[5] Timing is a key element distinguishing acute pain from subacute or chronic pain. Acute pain usually lasts up to 7 days but sometimes as long as 30 days. Chronic pain is defined as persistent or recurrent pain lasting longer than 3 months.[6] The 2019 National Health Interview Survey identified back, hip, knee, and foot pain as the most common locations of chronic pain.[7]

BURDEN OF DISEASE

Pain is a universal occurrence, but a subjective, individualized experience. Throughout the life span, pain, whether acute or chronic in nature, is one of the most frequent causes of health care visits, reasons for taking medications, and major causes of work disability.[8] A 2023 Centers for Disease Control and Prevention (CDC) analysis of data from the National Health Interview survey estimated that approximately 21% of adults in the United States had chronic pain and 7% of adults had high-impact chronic pain with substantial restriction of daily activities. The prevalence of chronic pain was higher in female individuals and may be more than 40% in older adults, with osteoarthritis and low back pain the most common etiologies.[8] The Institute of Medicine (IOM) acknowledged more than 100 million adults were impacted by persistent pain.[6]

Chronic pain has a plethora of psychosocial and socioeconomic impacts not only affecting individuals but also families and society. In 2010, the costs of chronic pain in the United States alone were estimated at more than US$560 billion due to direct medical costs, lost productivity, and disability programs (excluding cost of care for childcare, military personnel, institutionalized adults, and personal caregivers).[6] Individuals with chronic pain report significantly more missed workdays compared with those without chronic pain. Respondents also reported limitations in daily functioning, social activities, and activities of daily living.[7]

Unfortunately, disparities in consistent pain management across various racial and ethnic groups, gender, and socioeconomic status exist. These disparities, along with access to care with evidence-based pain treatments, prevent many people with pain from accessing the full range of potentially helpful therapies.[9] Using nationally representative data, Ly found significant racial and ethnic disparities in patient visit time with physicians and receipt of opioids for pain in the outpatient setting.[10] Specifically, Hispanic patients had shorter visits for back pain than White patients and both Black and Hispanic patients were less likely than White patients to receive opioids for abdominal and back pain. Hispanic patients were also more likely than White patients to receive nonopioids in lieu of opioids for both abdominal pain and back pain.[9] Among Black and White patients receiving opioids for pain, Black patients were less likely to be referred to a pain specialist, and Black patients received prescription opioids at lower dosages than White patients.[10–12] Geographic location also existed as a disparity leading to the increased use of opioids for conditions for which nonopioid treatment options may be preferred, but less available. Dowell and colleagues reported that adults living in rural areas were more likely to be prescribed opioids for chronic nonmalignant pain than adults living in nonrural areas.[10–12]

TREATMENT GOALS

Despite the opioid epidemic, inadequate treatment of pain must not only be assessed but addressed by health care providers. One of the most critical goals in pain management is the assurance and delivery of person-centered care, built on therapeutic and trusting relationships between the client and health care provider. Ideally, pain management is most successful with a multidisciplinary team approach. Pain management goals include improving pain control and function as well as enhancing coping skills to deal with ongoing pain.[13] Though a substantial part of pain care management occurs in the primary care setting, all clinicians providing patient care is responsible for keeping abreast on the therapeutic modalities, pharmacologic, alternative, and integrative alike. As advocates and gatekeepers, primary care providers must have knowledge of evidence-based guidelines and recommendations of pain management to provide the competent, holistic care and education clients deserve.

RECOMMENDATIONS

In 2022, the CDC released an updated clinical practice guideline for clinicians pre-scribing opioids to adult patients with pain, in outpatient settings. The guideline excluded care of pain in the setting of cancer, sickle cell disease, palliative care, or end-of-life care.[3] Twelve recommendations based on systematic reviews of the scien-tific literature, reflect risk/benefit considerations, patient and clinician value and pref-erences, and resource allocation. The CDC provides grades of the recommendations, category A or B and the type of evidence (1, 2, 3, or 4), based on the Advisory Com-mittee on Immunization Practice adapted grading of recommendations, assessment, development, and evaluation approach.[14] An overarching intention of the clinical prac-tice guideline was to improve patient/clinician communication regarding the risks and benefits of a variety of pain treatments, while also improving the safety and effective-ness of both pain mitigation and treatment, improving quality of life for individuals with pain, and reducing risks associated with opioid pain therapy such as opioid use dis-order, overdose, and death.[3]

For the sake of brevity, the 12 recommendations will be listed and summarized. The recommendations are grouped into 4 areas (**Box 1**) as well as 5 guiding principles to broadly inform implementation across recommendations (**Box 2**).

- Nonopioid therapies are at least as effective as opioids for many common types of acute pain. Nonpharmacologic and nonopioid pharmacologic therapies shall be maximized, as appropriate, for the specific condition and patient and only consider opioid therapy for acute pain if benefits are anticipated to outweigh risks to the patient. Realistic benefits and known risks of opioid therapy should be dis-cussed with patients prior to initiating opioid therapy for acute pain (recommen-dation category: B; evidence type: 3).
- Nonopioid therapies are preferred for subacute and chronic pain. Clinicians should maximize use of nonpharmacologic and nonopioid pharmacologic therapies as appropriate for the specific condition and patient and only consider initiating opioid therapy if expected benefits for pain and function are anticipated to outweigh risks to the patient. Before starting opioid therapy for subacute or chronic pain, clinicians should discuss with patients the realistic benefits and known risks of opioid ther-apy, should work with patients to establish treatment goals for pain and function, and should consider how opioid therapy will be discontinued if benefits do not outweigh risks (recommendation category: A; evidence type: 2).
- When starting opioid therapy for acute, subacute, or chronic pain, clinicians should prescribe immediate-release opioids instead of extended-release and long-acting (LA) opioids (recommendation category: A; evidence type: 4).

Box 1
Recommendation areas

1. Determining whether or not to initiate opioids for pain

2. Selecting opioids and appropriate dosing

3. Deciding duration of initial opioid prescription and conducting follow-up

4. Assessing risk and potential harms of opioid use

From Centers for Disease Control and Prevention. (2023). Clinical practice guideline for pre-scribing opioids for pain. U. S. Department of Health and Human Services. https://www.cdc.gov/mmwr/volumes/71/rr/rr7103a1.htm.

Box 2
Principles for implementation of recommendations areas

1. Regardless of whether opioids are part of a treatment regimen, acute, subacute, and chronic pain should be appropriately assessed and treated.

2. Recommendations are voluntary and flexible in order to support individualized, person-centered care, meeting the needs and circumstances of individual patients.

3. A multimodal and multidisciplinary approach to pain management that encompasses holistic care from the acute stage through long term is essential.

4. Special attention is warranted in order to avoid misapplying the clinical practice guideline beyond its intended use to prevent unintended and potentially harmful patient consequences.

5. All stakeholders should vigilantly attend to health inequities, providing culturally competent communication, ensuring appropriate affordable, diversified, and effective pharmacologic and nonpharmacologic pain management regimens for all individuals.

From Centers for Disease Control and Prevention. (2023). Clinical practice guideline for pre-scribing opioids for pain. U. S. Department of Health and Human Services. https://www.cdc.gov/mmwr/volumes/71/rr/rr7103a1.htm.

- When opioids are initiated for opioid-naïve patients with acute, subacute, or chronic pain, clinicians should prescribe the lowest effective dosage. If opioids are continued for subacute or chronic pain, clinicians should use caution when prescribing opioids at any dosage, should carefully evaluate individual benefits and risks when considering increasing dosage, and should avoid increasing dosage above levels likely to yield diminishing returns in benefits relative to risks to patients (recommendation category: A; evidence type: 3).
- For patients already receiving opioid therapy, clinicians should carefully weigh benefits and risks and exercise care when changing opioid dosage. If the benefits outweigh risks of continued opioid therapy, the patient and health care team should optimize implementation of nonopioid therapies into the plan of care. If benefits do not outweigh risks of continued opioid therapy, clinicians should optimize other therapies and work closely with patients to gradually taper to lower dosages or, if warranted based on the individual circumstances of the patient, appropriately taper and discontinue opioids. Unless there are indications of a life-threatening issue such as warning signs of impending overdose, opioid therapy should not be discontinued abruptly, and clinicians should not rapidly reduce opioid dosages from higher dosages (recommendation category: B; evidence type: 4).
- When opioids are needed for acute pain, clinicians should prescribe no greater quantity than needed for the expected duration of pain severe enough to require opioids (recommendation category: A; evidence type: 4).
- Clinicians should evaluate benefits and risks with patients within 1 to 4 weeks of starting opioid therapy for subacute or chronic pain or of dosage escalation. Clinicians should regularly re-evaluate benefits and risks of continued opioid therapy with patients (recommendation category: A; evidence type: 4).
- Before starting and periodically during continuation of opioid therapy, clinicians should evaluate risk for opioid-related harms and discuss risk with patients. Clinicians should work with patients to incorporate into the management plan

strategies to mitigate risk, including offering naloxone (recommendation category: A; evidence type: 4).

- When prescribing initial opioid therapy for acute, subacute, or chronic pain, and periodically during opioid therapy for chronic pain, clinicians should review the patient's history of controlled substance prescriptions using state prescription drug monitoring program data to determine whether the patient is receiving opioid dosages or combinations that put the patient at high risk for overdose (recommendation category: B; evidence type: 4).
- When prescribing opioids for subacute or chronic pain, clinicians should consider the benefits and risks of toxicology testing to assess for prescribed medications as well as other prescribed and nonprescribed controlled substances (recommendation category: B; evidence type: 4).
- Clinicians should use particular caution when prescribing opioid pain medication and benzodiazepines concurrently and consider whether benefits outweigh risks of concurrent prescribing of opioids and other central nervous system depressants (recommendation category: B; evidence type 3).
- Clinicians should offer or arrange treatment with evidence-based medications to treat patients with opioid use disorder. Detoxification on its own, without medications for opioid use disorder, is not recommended because of increased risks for resuming drug use, overdose, and overdose death (recommendation category: A; evidence type: 1).

NONPHARMACOLOGICAL MANAGEMENT

Noninvasive nonpharmacologic approaches to acute pain have the potential to improve pain and function without risk for serious harms. Nonpharmacologic therapies (ice, heat, elevation, rest, immobilization, or exercise) should be maximized, as appropriate, for specific conditions. A variety of noninvasive nonpharmacologic approaches include heat therapy for low back pain; spinal manipulation for acute back pain with radiculopathy; a cervical collar or exercise for acute neck pain with radiculopathy; acupressure for acute musculoskeletal pain; massage for postoperative pain; and electrical neuromodulation for acute pain related to episodic migraines.[3] Therapeutics to lessen pain and promote soft tissue healing, include stretching, strengthening, and endurance exercise such as yoga, have been found to improve nonspecific back pain. Physical modalities via heat and cold produce thermal tissue changes, at least temporarily relieving pain.[13] The American College of Physicians (ACP) and the American Association of Family Physicians (AAFP) discuss a plethora of nonpharmacologic therapies to reduce pain ranging from acupressure, transcutaneous electrical nerve stimulation, joint manipulation therapy, exercise, education, and mobilization to name a few. The aforementioned recommendations range from high to low certainty of evidence based on the literature.[15]

Though evidence supports the use of noninvasive nonpharmacologic therapies, access and cost can be barriers as many insurances fail to cover alternative modalities as well as disparities for those who are uninsured, have limited income, transportation challenges, or live in rural areas where alternative treatments are not available.

MEDICAL AND PHARMACOLOGIC MANAGEMENT

The literature supports nonopioid therapies are at least as effective as opioids for common acute pain conditions, including low back pain, neck pain, musculoskeletal injuries, pain secondary to minor surgeries and postoperative pain associated with minimal tissue injury as well as dental pain, kidney stone pain, and headaches including episodic migraine.[3] Nonopioid pharmacologics (topical or oral nonsteroidal anti-inflammatory drugs [NSAIDs], acetaminophen) and nonpharmacologic therapies (ice, heat, elevation, rest, immobilization, or exercise) should be maximized, as appropriate, for specific conditions.[3] The ACP and AAFP recommend treatment of acute pain from non-low back, musculoskeletal injuries with topical NSAIDs with or without menthol gel as first-line therapy to reduce or relieve pain, improve physical function, and improve patient's treatment satisfaction.[15] NSAIDs are first-line drug of choice if medically appropriate while duloxetine, tricyclic antidepressants, or rare use of tramadol are considered second-line drug therapy for chronic musculoskeletal pain.[13] For those patients experiencing neuropathic pain, such as diabetic neuropathy, sciatica, postherpetic neuralgia, spinal arachnoiditis, and phantom limb pain, first-line pharmacologic therapies should focus on membrane-stabilizing medications such as gabapentin, pregabalin, duloxetine, tricyclic antidepressants, and topical local anesthetics.[13]

Opioid therapy does play an important role for acute pain associated with severe traumatic injuries such as crush injuries, burns, invasive surgeries associated with moderate-to-severe postoperative pain, and other severe acute pain when NSAIDs and other therapies are ineffective or contraindicated. When diagnosis and severity of acute pain warrant the use of opioids, clinicians should prescribe immediate-release opioids at the lowest effective dose for no longer than the expected duration of pain severe enough to require opioids. Opioids should be prescribed and used on an as-needed basis rather than on a scheduled basis.[3]

Clinicians have an important role in providing informed consent to patients to assure awareness of expected benefits, common and serious risks, and alternatives to opioids before starting and/or continuing opioid therapy.[3] While evidence does support short-term pain relief with opioid therapy, there is no difference in function, sleep, or mood. The literature does not provide a universally accepted safe dose of opioids. Additionally, the use of LA opioids and mixing other central nervous system depressants, such as benzodiazepines or alcohol, and carisoprodol, synergistically increases the risk of accidental lethal overdose.[13]

SUMMARY

Health disparities, supporting evidence, and limited access are only a few of the implications preventing holistic pain management to the millions of individuals affected by pain. Pain impacts millions of Americans, potentially reducing their level of function, mental health, and quality of life. Despite evidence that benefits of short-term pain relief are minimal with limited evidence of long-term benefits, opioids continue to be used for the management of acute and chronic pain.[9] Pain is a universal occurrence experienced by all individuals. Clinicians must be well-versed in evidence-based guidelines to provide both competence and confidence clients deserve for successful pain management.

CLINICS CARE POINTS

- Throughout history, one of the greatest medical challenges involves the conundrum of treating pain. Pain management has and continues to be a long-standing public health concern.

- Young, White men in rural Appalachia with low levels of education, employment, and mental health disorders are among those at highest risk for substance use and overdose.[1]

- Pain is a universal occurrence, but a subjective, individualized experience.

- Chronic pain has a plethora of psychosocial and socioeconomic impacts not only affecting individuals but also families and society.
- Clinicians should strive to develop trusting, therapeutic relationships with clients to provide compassionate, holistic, and appropriate care to individuals with pain.
- Nonopioid therapies are preferred for subacute and chronic pain.
- The literature supports nonopioid therapies are at least as effective as opioids for common acute pain conditions, including low back pain, neck pain, musculoskeletal injuries, pain secondary to minor surgeries and postoperative pain associated with minimal tissue injury as well as dental pain, kidney stone pain, and headaches including episodic migraine.[3]
- Clinicians must be well-versed in evidence-based guidelines to provide both competence and confidence clients deserve for successful pain management.

DISCLOSURE

The author has nothing to disclose.

REFERENCES

1. Schalkoff C, Lancaster K, Gaynes B, et al. The opioid and related drug epidemics in rural Appalachia: a systematic review of populations affected, risk factors, and infectious diseases. Subst Abuse 2020;41(1):35–69.
2. Buer L. Rx Appalachia: stories of treatment and survival in rural Kentucky. Chicago, IL: Haymarket Books; 2020.
3. Centers for Disease Control and Prevention. Clinical practice guideline for prescribing opioids for pain. U. S. Department of Health and Human Services; 2023. Available at: https://www.cdc.gov/mmwr/volumes/71/rr/rr7103a1.htm.
4. Raja SN, Carr DB, Cohen M, et al. The revised international association for the study of pain definition of pain Concepts, challenges, and compromises. Pain 2020;161(9):1976–82.
5. Tighe P, Buckenmaier CC 3rd, AP Boezaart, et al. Acute pain medicine in the United States: a status report. Pain Med 2015 Sep;16(9):1806–26.
6. Tauben D, Stacey B. Evaluation of chronic non-cancer pain in adults. Retrieved from UpToDate; 2023.
7. Institute of Medicine. Relieving pain in America: a Blueprint for Transforming prevention, care, education, and Research. Washington, DC: The National Academies Press; 2011.
8. Young RJ, Mullins PM, Bhattacharyya N. Prevalence of chronic pain among adults in the United States. Pain 2022;163(2):e328–32.
9. Dowell D, Ragan K, Jones C, et al. Prescribing opioids for pain-The new CDC clinical practice guideline. N Engl J Med 2022;387(22). Available at: https://www.nejm.org/doi/full/10.1056/NEJMp2211040.
10. Ly D. Racial and ethnic disparities in the evaluation and management of pain in the outpatient setting, 2006-2015. Pain Med 2022;20:223–32.
11. Morden N, Chyn D, Wood A, et al. Racial inequality in prescription opioid receipt-Role of individual health systems. N Engl J Med 2021;385:342–51.
12. Dowell D, Ragan KR, Jones CM, et al. Center for Disease Control Clinical practice guideline for prescribing opioids for pain-United States, 2022. MMWR Recomm Rep (Morb Mortal Wkly Rep) 2022;71(RR-3):1–95.

13. Owen G, Bruel B, Schrade C, et al. Pain medicine for primary care physicians. PROC-Baylor University Medical Center 2018;31(1):37–47.
14. Granholm A, Alhazzani W, Møller MH. Use of the GRADE approach in systematic reviews and guidelines. Br J Anaesth 2020;123(5):554–9.
15. Qaseem A, McLean R, Gurek D, et al, Clinical Guidelines Committee of the American College of Physicians. Nonpharmacologic and pharmacologic management of acute pain from non-low back, musculoskeletal injuries in adults: a clinical guideline from the American College of physicians and American Academy of family physicians. Ann Intern Med 2020;173(9):739–48.

Navigating Pediatric Pain
Emerging Trends and Best Practice

Debra Sullivan, PhD, MSN, RN, CNE, COI*, Christine Frazer, PhD, CNS, CNE

KEYWORDS

- Pediatric pain • SDOH • Nurse perceptions • Nursing education • Assessment

KEY POINTS

- Nurses form therapeutic relationships with pediatric patients and their families, providing valuable insights into the child's pain experience.
- Education and training are necessary to keep current and future acute care pediatric nurses abreast of the assessment and management of pediatric pain.
- Nurses must evaluate parents and one's own perceptions, beliefs, and biases that can hinder assessing and managing children's pain.
- Pediatric pain management is holistic in assessing pain with validated tools, recognizing developmental factors, and social determinants of health in treatment involving families and an interdisciplinary team. Treatment uses pharmacologic and non-pharmacologic interventions for multimodal therapies.
- Nurses blend clinical skills and emotional intelligence while considering child development levels to assess and manage pediatric pain.

INTRODUCTION

This article explores nurses' crucial role in pediatric pain management, including nurse education and training, accurate pain assessment, and pharmacologic and non-pharmacologic approaches, and offering emotional support to empower patients and families with knowledge. The challenges and opportunities nurses encounter in this field, current pain management practices, and the need for more precise and personalized care are presented.

In the scope of pediatric care, effective pain management holds paramount importance, as it directly impacts the well-being and quality of life of young patients. Children, with their unique developmental characteristics and varied pain experiences, require specialized care that addresses not only the physical aspects of pain but also the emotional and psychological dimensions.[1] Those in intensive care units experience high levels of pain and anxiety[2,3] that are often undertreated.[4] Nurses, as

College of Nursing, Walden University, 100 Washington Avenue South, Suite 1210, Minneapolis, MN 55401, USA
* Corresponding author.
E-mail address: Debra.sullivan@mail.waldenu.edu

Crit Care Nurs Clin N Am 36 (2024) 479–494
https://doi.org/10.1016/j.cnc.2024.04.004
0899-5885/24/© 2024 Elsevier Inc. All rights reserved.

frontline caregivers, play a pivotal role in orchestrating comprehensive and compassionate approaches to pediatric pain management. Their expertise in assessing, intervening, and advocating for pediatric patients ensures that pain is not only alleviated but also understood and managed in a manner that respects the individuality of each child.[4]

Pediatric pain management extends far beyond the administration of analgesics.[5] It involves a dynamic blend of clinical skills, emotional intelligence, and a deep understanding of child development. Nurses have the privilege of forming therapeutic relationships with young patients and their families, which provides them with valuable insights into the child's pain experience.[4,6] This insight is central to devising tailored pain management plans that address not only the physical discomfort but also the potential anxiety, fear, and uncertainty that often accompany pain in children.[7,8]

As advocates for their patients, acute care nurses contribute to a comprehensive approach to pediatric pain management that extends to collaboration with other health care team members,[9] clear communication with families, consideration of social determinants of health (SDOH),[10] and active involvement in pain education.[11] Ultimately, this article underscores how nursing care in the context of pediatric pain management is not only about addressing physical discomfort but also about nurturing trust, instilling confidence, and promoting a sense of control for both young patients and their caregivers. The acute care nurse must navigate this intricate landscape of pediatric pain management, where nursing expertise and compassionate care converge to create a brighter, more comfortable journey for young patients facing pain challenges.

In this article, nurses' crucial role in pediatric pain management is explored, including nurse education and training, accurate pain assessment, and pharmacologic and non-pharmacologic approaches, and offering emotional support to empower both patients and families with knowledge. The challenges and opportunities nurses encounter in this field, current pain management practices, and the need for more precise and personalized care are presented.

BACKGROUND
Pediatric Pain: Nursing Education and Training

Globally, pediatric pain is a challenge and is often inadequately assessed, undertreated, and mismanaged.[12–19] The American Nurses Association (ANA)[20] standards maintain that nurses are responsible for providing optimal care to persons experiencing pain and, ethically, to relieve pain. Facilitating current and future nurse competency in pain management is warranted[16] as a knowledge-to-practice gap continues to remain.[18,19] The ANA[20] supports ongoing education to help maintain and support nurse competency in pain management. Inasmuch, organizations that offer in-services on a routine basis help to keep pain management front and center as a priority.[13,21]

In undergraduate education, it is imperative for student nurses to acquire competencies associated with pain management across the lifespan and application in clinical practice before graduation.[17] Competent faculty members who are experienced and possess sound knowledge to teach pain content throughout the lifespan, specifically as it relates to the pediatric population, are necessary.[17] Faculty at academic institutions should keep abreast of best practices toward pain management and routinely review and update pain curricula, lessons, and instructional strategies, and evaluate student achievement of learning outcomes.[16] Transformative learning in the educational setting is valuable. Role-playing, simulations, and other methods can effectively promote self-reflection, gain a new perspective, and deepen student awareness.[22] Moreover, the learning process becomes more engaging and meaningful to students, and it can help to expand critical thinking skills.[22] Beyond the classroom environment, taking a transformational approach to clinical experiences is worthy of consideration—for example, arranging clinical experiences in homeless shelters, halfway houses, and with specialized pediatric non-profit organizations like the National Pediatric Cancer Foundation and Autism Spectrum Disorder Foundation. Lastly, educators should look to collaborate with expert pediatric clinicians in the field and invite opportunities to share pediatric care components and resources with students.[22]

Nurses must possess the knowledge and skills necessary to adequately address, assess, and effectively manage pediatric pain. Successfully managing pain can positively influence numerous factors, such as the healing process, mobilization, hospital length of stay, and overall cost associated with care and treatment.[18] A deficiency in nursing knowledge ultimately hinders outcomes of effective pain management[20] as nurses become reluctant to initiate interventions secondary to their lack of confidence.[14]

Nursing education, training, and in-service opportunities not only enhance pediatric pain management competencies but can also help to demystify any potential misconceptions, myths, biases, and stigmas associated with managing pediatric pain.[16,23] Preconceived biases and prejudices can potentially influence the pain management approach.[6,10] Thus, nursing students, as well as current health care providers, must explore their own experiences, backgrounds, values, and beliefs surrounding pain to "set aside or bracket their biases so they can better understand the patient's experience."[20]

PAIN MANAGEMENT APPROACHES
Assessment

Acute care nurses have the challenging task of assessing pain in children of different ages, developmental stages, and acuity levels,[24] and more so when an infant or young child cannot verbalize or confirm their pain.[25] To promote optimal management of pain, improved outcomes, and prevention of unnecessary discomfort, it is imperative to accurately assess pain early and often.[26,27] Furthermore, to build an atmosphere of a supportive environment, nurses should involve the child and parents in the assessment of pain.[13,25]

Assessing pediatric pain can be particularly difficult because routine assessments tend to focus on behavioral and physiologic factors.[24] Behavioral factors include observable reactions such as vocalizations (ie, crying, moaning), head shaking, drawing up knees, or facial expressions (ie, grimacing). In contrast, physiologic factors involve changes in vital signs, such as increased heart rate or blood pressure or a shift in respiratory rate and pattern.[24,28] Pain increases the stress response, which, in turn, can further impact oral intake, gastric emptying, and, for some, cause nausea and vomiting.[29] While these factors are necessary to assess and further guide pain management, SDOH and essential components, such as past experiences, perceptions, beliefs, biases, cultural differences, and stereotypes, are oftentimes overlooked. Nurses must examine SDOH and other essential components to provide the best possible care. Additionally, a comprehensive understanding of these factors' influence on pediatric pain assessment and management is crucial to optimizing patient outcomes.

Pediatric Pain Management Approach: Assessment of Social Determinants of Health and Other Essential Factors

The World Health Organization[30] defines SDOH as non-medical factors that influence health outcomes such as age and where individuals are born, live, work, and the forces and systems affecting the daily conditions of life. The five domains that encompass SDOH include economic stability, access to quality education, quality health care, neighborhood and built environment, and social and community context. Child health outcomes are greatly influenced by SDOH and the encompassing domains.[31,32] For instance, children living in poverty are frequently exposed to environments characterized by high levels of crime and violence, limited transportation options, and scarce access to quality education, modern and state-of-the-art medical facilities, and experienced health care professionals.[33,34] This has a direct impact on children and their basic human needs, thus influencing their overall quality of life and health status, placing them at a higher risk for illness and other social disparities.[33] Developing a child's physical, social, and emotional capabilities is foundational to their health and wellness.[31] In a recent study conducted by Xiao and colleagues,[35] children who were socioeconomically deprived experienced the worst outcomes in comparison to children in other SDOH categories. As well, Andrist and colleagues[32] research points to a correlation that exists between neighborhood poverty, poor health outcomes, and a child's need for pediatric intensive care. Therefore, with nearly half of the children in America living in low-income households,[36] screening for SDOH factors is a proactive approach toward improving health outcomes and an important first step toward gaining insight into disparities that can affect current and future health outcomes.[33,35]

Although plenty of health-related screening tools exist, a limited number apply to health-related social conditions and pediatrics or family practice.[37] Currently, the American Association of Pediatrics[38] houses a collection of screening tools on various topics, including those related to social drivers of health. Some examples are the Protocol for Responding to and Assessing Patients Assets, Risks, and Experiences (PRAPARE), A Safe Environment for Every Kid (SEEK) Questionnaire, Well Child Care, Evaluation, Community Resources, Advocacy, Referral, Education (WE CARE), Children's HealthWatch Survey, and the Hunger Vital Sign tool. Given the impact of SDOH factors on a child's current and future health outcomes, future development of screening tools is warranted. At the forefront, nurses play a vital role in assessing for SDOH and connecting patients and families to the resources.[29,39] As a whole, the health care lens must continue to evolve and become increasingly in-tuned toward the cultural, social, economic, and environmental conditions that exist to obtain the highest possible standard of optimal health for all.

Perceptions: Influences on Beliefs, Stereotypes, and Biases

In addition to assessing SDOH, examining the association between perceptions and their influence on beliefs, stereotypes, and biases surrounding pain is also crucial. First, it is essential to note that perceptions and experiences regarding pain are unique to each individual.[26] For instance, what one person may consider mild pain, another may perceive as severe. Research points to the significant impact past experiences with pain can have on perceptions, future pain, and outcomes.[40,41] Untreated pain related to procedures (ie, needle sticks to start an IV or venipuncture for blood draws) can lead to a future fear of needles.[41,42] Undertreatment of pain can impact seeking future health care.[41,42] Moreover, pain that is mismanaged or undertreated may delay recovery, potentiate complications, and ultimately impact the length of stay.[13,40,43] Therefore, nurses must assess past experiences and consider them when evaluating and managing a child's current pain.

Equally important is the necessity to gain insight into beliefs founded on myths or misconceptions about pain.[44,45] It is not uncommon for pain to be misconstrued by parents and nurses, especially when it comes to children and their vocalization of pain or lack thereof. For instance, when children are quiet and appear resting, pain is often perceived as non-existent.[13,44,46] However, a conviction also exists that when it comes to pain, children often overreport.[44] Nurses' misconceptions about pain often stem from factors such as lack of work experience, education, and training.[13,46] Therefore, addressing misconceptions is crucial to ensure children receive adequate pain management.

Additionally, research identified parent hesitation toward the use of analgesics for managing children's pain due to unfounded fears related to adverse effects and potential addiction.[45,46] In Yu and Kim's[46] study surrounding Hispanic and Korean families, parents of girls feared side effects associated with pharmaceuticals the most. However, Hispanic and Korean parents of boys expressed even greater fear and desired boys to avoid medications so they could be tougher within their culture.[46] Similar to parents and their beliefs, nurse beliefs and misconceptions also play a part in overestimating the risk of addiction when considering the administration of opioid analgesics to children.[47] Thus, fears and erroneous beliefs about addictions can significantly hinder effective pain management and optimal pain relief for children.[45,47]

Biases and stereotypes associated with race, gender, and ethnicity can have a significant impact on how pediatric pain is perceived and influence the overall course of actions to take when it comes to pediatric pain management.[48,49] Biases can influence provider attitudes and actions.[48,49] In association with race, for example, a study by Sabin and colleagues[50] using vignettes found that providers who highly favored Whites were less likely to prescribe opioids to African American children for the management of post-surgical pain. Similarly, minority children in outpatient visits were less likely to receive opioids for pain management versus Whites.[51] Furthermore, biases are also prevalent when it comes to gender and pediatric perceptions of pain and its management. For instance, in comparison to boys, others perceive girls as more sensitive to pain and more expressive when it comes to their pain experiences.[52] However, there's a concerning tendency to underestimate or dismiss girls' pain experiences based on these very stereotypes.[52–54] More recently, when male and female patients reported the same level of pain and expressiveness,[55] perceivers continued to discredit and underestimate pain experienced in females and overestimated men and their self-report of pain. Thus, gender bias and pain stereotypes continue to exist. Lastly, study findings revealed ethnic disparities and biases associated with pediatric children and the management of their pain. Specifically, when presenting with severe pain, Hispanic and Black Non-Hispanic (NH) children were less likely to be administered opioid analgesia compared to White NH children who received an opioid when experiencing the same amount of pain.[56]

Various factors can play a role in influencing pediatric pain, including child age, developmental stage, cultural upbringing, coping strategies, mood, as well as current and past experiences of pain.[17,19] Therefore, creating and effectively instituting an individualized approach to child pain assessment and management is best practice.[26] Nurses and the health care team can better understand pediatric pain by conducting frequent, detailed, and personalized evaluations and closely analyzing SDOH and other factors influencing pediatric pain, such as perceptions and their impact on beliefs, stereotypes, and biases. This practice can lead to an improvement in the overall management of pain in children.

Plan

Pediatric pain management is a critical aspect of health care aimed at alleviating pain and improving the quality of life for children and adolescents. Pain that is managed poorly in children or uncontrolled pain can lead to chronic pain, distress, anxiety, and disability in adulthood.[26,57] The experience of pain in the pediatric population is complex influenced by developmental stages, cognitive capacities, SDOH, and emotional well-being.[57] Effective pain management strategies for this population encompass a holistic approach, integrating pharmacologic and non-pharmacologic interventions alongside advanced pain assessment tools. This section delves into the multifaceted realm of pediatric pain management, exploring the evolving landscape of approaches that seek to minimize pain and enhance the well-being of young patients.

Pharmacologic Approaches to Pediatric Pain Management

Pharmacologic interventions play a pivotal role in managing pediatric pain, providing relief across a spectrum of acute and chronic conditions. Over the years, advancements in pediatric pharmacology have led to more tailored and precise medication regimens, minimizing adverse effects and optimizing efficacy. These approaches include the use of analgesics, opioids, local anesthetics, and adjuvant medications, all of which are dosed and administered based on factors such as age, weight, and the nature of the pain.[26,58,59]

Opioid agents are the cornerstone of treating pediatric acute pain.[9] According to a scoping review in 2019, the most common pharmacologic agents used to manage pain in the intensive care unit (ICU) were opioids.[7] Morphine is one of the most widely used and, with accepted dosing recommendations, has been safe and effective in children. Neonates and infants receive a more conservative dosing.[59] Other opioids used are fentanyl, oxycodone, hydromorphone, codeine, tramadol, and tapentadol[59] **(Table 1)**.

Pharmacokinetics examines how the body interacts with medication doses during exposure, while pharmacodynamics studies the drugs' effects on the body.[60] During childhood, the pharmacokinetics in all medications change due to body size and renal and metabolic drug clearance maturation.[59] Another issue is that the initial and maintenance dosing using pharmacokinetic parameters is based on volume and clearance. Still, the commonly used "dose per kilogram" can underdose due to only considering volume based on weight and not drug clearance pathways.[59] Pharmacodynamics has not been well studied in infants or children; however, it has been accepted that infants are pharmacodynamically immature and sensitive to opioid concentrations, showing a reduced clearance rate of 10% to 20% compared to older children.[59]

Table 1 Opioids and administration	
Opioid	**Available Routes**
Morphine	IV, NCA/PCA infusion, PO
Fentanyl	IV bolus, NCA/PCA bolus, NCA infusion
Oxycodone	IV bolus, PO
Hydromorphone	IV bolus, NCA/PCA bolus, NCA infusion
Tramadol	IV bolus, PO
Tapentadol	PO

Abbreviations: IV, intravenous; NCA, nurse-controlled analgesia; PCA, patient-controlled analgesia; PO, per oris.

Adapted from Aziznejadroshan P, Alhani F, Mohammadi E. Experience of nurses about barriers to pain management in pediatric units: A qualitative study. J Nurs Midwifery Sci. 2017;4(3):89. https://doi.org/10.4103/JNMS.JNMS_2_17.

Also reported in the scoping review were other lesser-used medications used for pain management in the pediatric intensive care unit (PICU): remifentanil, dexmedetomidine, acetaminophen, ketorolac, lidocaine (local anesthetic), bupivacaine (regional anesthetic),[7] and non-steroidal anti-inflammatories.[58] One study, with a sample size of 984 pediatric units from 390 hospitals, found that PICUs used pharmacologic pain interventions 78.2% of the time compared to non-pharmacologic interventions.[58] Pharmacologic agents are heavily used in the critical care unit (CCU); however, nurses should be aware of multimodal and non-pharmacologic methods as adjuncts to pain management.

Multidisciplinary analgesia treatments must be considered for the critical care patient due to the potential for adverse outcomes related to opioid use.[9] Opioids have several adverse side effects, including respiratory depression, constipation, cognitive dysfunction, and psychiatric issues.[9] Multimodal treatment uses multiple medications for pain management and is considered optimal for acute pain management. Opioid-sparing adjuvants targeting specific pain physiology include nociceptive (acetaminophen, non-steroidal anti-inflammatories, and glucocorticoids) and neuropathic medication (gabapentinoids, lidocaine, ketamine, and alpha 2 agonist).[9] Other multidisciplinary enhancements to pain management could include a child life specialist, a child psychologist, and behavioral pain management interventions.

Non-pharmacologic Approaches to Pediatric Pain Management

In recognition of the need for well-rounded pain management, non-pharmacologic interventions have gained prominence in pediatric care. These approaches encompass various techniques that target psychological, physical, and environmental factors contributing to pain. Techniques such as distraction therapy, deep breathing relaxation exercises, music therapy, art therapy, mindfulness, medical hypnosis, and virtual reality interventions engage the young patients' senses and divert their attention from the pain stimulus.[7,9] These methods complement pharmacologic interventions and offer patients a sense of control and empowerment in managing their pain.

The most common non-pharmacologic pain interventions found in a large study of critical care nurses were distraction, relaxation, music, repositioning, and environment modification.[58] In another study that looked at 224 nurses who worked in 16 ICUs across northern Iran, the researchers found that 55.8% of the nurses used non-pharmacologic interventions for pain.[61] The most common method was repositioning, using comfort equipment, and providing a quiet and comfortable room.[61]

Critical care nurses play a vital role in multimodal pain management, but a lack of training in non-pharmacological interventions can be a barrier.[15] When using a multidisciplinary approach, child life specialists and child psychologists can support non-pharmaceutical treatments in the CCU.[9] The use of non-pharmacologic pain management has been shown to reduce pain, decrease opioid use, and decrease the length of hospital stay.[9,62]

Pediatric Pain Assessment Tools

Accurate assessment of pediatric pain is complex but crucial for tailoring appropriate interventions.[7] However, the subjective nature of pain perception can pose challenges in accurately gauging a child's pain experience. Pain assessment in the CCU includes physiologic, psychological, behavioral, social, SDOH, and developmental factors. Other factors to consider are the critical nature of the child's illness and their ability to communicate.[7] To address these variables, several pain assessment tools have been developed, taking into account the child's age, cognitive development, and communication abilities. See **Table 2** for a list of common pediatric pain tools. These

Table 2
Pediatric pain assessment tools

Tool	Comment	Reference
Wong-Baker FACES Pain Rating Scale	Widely used for ages 3 and older	©1983 Wong-Baker FACES Foundation. www.WongBakerFACES.org
FLACC (Face, Legs, Activity, Cry, Controllability Scale)	The Behavioral Pain Assessment Scale is used for non-verbal or preverbal patients. Commonly used in pediatric ICU.	Merkel S, Voepel-Lewis T, Shayevitz JR, et al. The FLACC: A behavioural scale for scoring postoperative pain in young children. Pediatric nursing 1997; 23:293-797.
CRIES	Used for infants >38 wk gestation	Krechel SW, Bildner J. CRIES: a new neonatal postoperative pain measurement score. Initial testing of validity and reliability. Paediatr Anaesth. 1995;5(1):53–61. https://doi.org/10.1111/j.1460-9592.1995.tb00242.x
N-Pass	Neonatal Pain Agitation and Sedation Scale	Hummel PA, Puchalski ML, Creech SD, Weiss MG: N-PASS: Neonatal Pain, Agitation and Sedation Scale-Reliability and Validity. J Perinatology 2008;28:55–60.
Oucher	2 scales: 0–100 numeric and 6 picture photographic scale	Beyer JE, Denyes MJ, Villarruel AM. The creation, validation, and continuing development of the Oucher: a measure of pain intensity in children. J Pediatr Nurs. 1992;7(5):335–346.
Numeric or Visual Analog Scales	There are many available	

tools enable health care providers to comprehend the child's pain experience better, facilitating more personalized and effective treatment plans. According to a large study, the most common tool used for pediatric pain assessment in PICUs was the face, legs, activity, cry, consolability (FLACC) scale, which is a behavioral pain assessment tool for non-verbal or preverbal patients.[58]

Holistic Approach and Future Directions

Critical care nurses must approach pediatric pain management with a holistic approach that recognizes the interconnectedness of physical, emotional, and psychological well-being. A collaborative effort involving health care professionals, parents, and young patients is essential for successful pain management. Furthermore, ongoing research aims to refine existing approaches and explore innovative techniques, such as the use of personalized medicine, to enhance pediatric pain management outcomes further.

BARRIERS

Nurses are morally and professionally responsible for managing pediatric pain, including assessment, administering analgesics, and using other non-pharmaceutical methods to ease pain.[15] However, nurses experience barriers to managing pediatric pain due to unique challenges in the patient population they care for, such as the patient's developmental level, cognitive development, communication abilities, parental involvement, SDOH, fear and anxiety, and fear of addiction.[1,5,15,61] Not only are difficulties on the patient side, but there are also barriers from the nurse's perspective, such as the nurse's knowledge of analgesics, reluctance to administer pain medication due to fear of overdosing, lack of time, nurse fatigue, heavy workload, staff shortages, working pressure, and organizational culture in general.[1,5,15,61] In the PICU, there are additional challenges in providing pain management, such as the complexity of the critical condition, the intensity of emotions in this environment, sedative agents, mechanical ventilation, and the patient's level of consciousness.[1]

A multidisciplinary approach involving health care providers, parents, psychologists, and pain specialists is crucial to overcome these barriers. Tailoring pain management strategies to the child's developmental stage, cultural considerations, communication abilities, and specific medical conditions is essential for effective and compassionate care.[9] Ongoing disparities in pain management for children from underserved communities are due to SDOH, such as race and ethnicity.[10] In a large study looking at racial and ethnic differences in pain management in pediatric patients, it was found that minority children were less likely to receive opioids and did not experience optimal pain reduction.[10]

Parental understanding of pediatric pain management strategies can vary. Lack of awareness or misinformation about available treatment options could impact the child's pain relief, especially when parents play a critical role in pain management.[15,63] In a descriptive study, parents of children who had acute pain reported satisfaction with the pain management service and showed adequate knowledge of pediatric pain. However, there were incongruencies between the intensity of "pain, satisfaction on the adequacy of pain management and knowledge and attitudes."[63] Ethical issues can arise when the child's wishes differ from those of their parents or guardians. Critical care nurses must navigate these complex situations to uphold the child's best interests.

Organizational culture and structure can also be barriers to pain management. Nurses have reported staff shortages, lack of time, excessive workload, and lack of physician support.[1,5,15] Critical care nurses may lack adequate training in pediatric pain management, resulting in suboptimal pain assessment and treatment. To effectively approach solutions to these barriers, collaboration with a multidisciplinary team is needed to develop policies and protocols to prioritize pain management for evidence-based pain assessment and appropriate pharmacologic and nonpharmacologic treatments.

These barriers highlight the ongoing complexities in pediatric pain management. Addressing these challenges requires a comprehensive approach encompassing medical, psychological, social, and ethical dimensions and collaboration among health care providers, parents, and other stakeholders.

CASE STUDY

Isabella, a 9-year-old Hispanic girl, was riding her bicycle to school from home, an apartment where she and her two younger siblings live with their parents. While nearing the intersection at the corner, Isabella was struck by a vehicle speeding through a red light at the crosswalk. She was airlifted 25 miles away to the closest trauma hospital. Following emergency surgery to repair a ruptured spleen, right lobe liver injury (grade V), and an open compound fracture of the ankle with exposed tibia, Isabella

Table 3
Case study

Nursing Action	Findings
Assessment	• The nurse entered Isabella's room to assess her pain. She uses a combination of behavioral indicators, such as facial expressions, body movements, and physiologic parameters. The nurse observes Isabella grimacing with a slight movement of the lower extremity and palpation of the abdomen. A numeric rating scale was used to assist in self-reported pain, and the FLACC scale was used to evaluate behavioral signs of pain. Isabella rates her pain at a 7 and verbalizes in English, "My belly hurts when I have to cough, and so does my leg." Vitals show heart rate and blood pressure elevated within the last hour. SpO_2 of 98%. There are no signs of bleeding at the surgical site and no hematuria. Fluid intake and output are adequate. • Isabella's parents are present in the room. The father speaks minimal English and responds by nodding and stating only no or yes. The mother replies to health professionals' questions with 2–3 words in English. The primary language for parents is Spanish. • To identify Isabella's and her family's strengths, challenges, and potential barriers, screening tools in her native language are utilized to evaluate social drivers of health (PRAPARE, SEEK Questionnaire, WE CARE, and Hunger Vital Sign tool).
Nursing Diagnosis	• Acute pain related to surgical incisions and abdominal and lower extremity discomfort as evidenced by clinical signs. • Impaired verbal communication related to language barrier as evidenced by non-English speaking parents. • Knowledge deficit related to available community support and available resources.
Nursing Interventions	Pain Management: • Medication: Isabella is prescribed pain medications suitable for her age and condition, such as IV acetaminophen and opioids. The doses are calculated based on her weight and adjusted to achieve optimal pain relief while minimizing side effects. • Multimodal Approach: The team uses a multimodal approach by combining medications with non-pharmacological interventions such as distraction techniques, music therapy, and comfort measures to reduce Isabella's perception of pain. • Positioning and Care: Isabella's nurse ensures she is comfortably positioned and her surgical site well-supported. Regular repositioning helps prevent pressure ulcers and discomfort. Parent Involvement • Keep Isabella's family informed about her progress, treatment plan, and any changes in her condition. • Encourage family involvement in Isabella's care routine such as assisting with breathing and ROM exercises, monitoring child pain, and providing comfort measures. • Provide educational material and visuals in Spanish. Utilize language apps or other communication devices to assist with translating when interpreter is not available. • Encourage parents to ask questions and express concerns. • Regular Assessment: Nurse consistently assesses Isabella's pain level and response to interventions. Adjustments are made based on Isabella's condition and feedback from the team.

(continued on next page)

Table 3 (continued)	
Nursing Action	**Findings**
	Emotional Support
	• Use child-friendly communication techniques to explain procedures, medications, and interventions to Isabella.
	• Offer emotional support to Isabella and her family, addressing their concerns and fears about her condition and care.
	Multidisciplinary Team
	• Child life specialist
	• Physical therapist
	• Physician
	• Nurses
	• Practitioners
	• Clinical nurse specialist
	• Social worker
	The multidisciplinary team works together to connect the family to available resources within the community regarding transportation support, future home health needs, financial assistance, food services, and other resources as needed.
Evaluation	• Continuously monitor Isabella's vital signs.
	• Assess pain level and response to pain management interventions.
	• Collaborate with the medical team to address any changes in Isabella's condition and adjust the treatment plan accordingly.
	• Communicate with Isabella's family to gather feedback on her comfort, emotional well-being, and overall care experience.
Communication and Documentation	The ICU team communicates Isabella's plan of care during shift handoffs to ensure continuity of care. Detailed documentation includes pain assessments, interventions administered, Isabella's response to treatment, positioning measures, assessment of incision, and parents' involvement with care.
Outcome	Over the course of Isabella's stay in the ICU, her pain is effectively managed. Her physiologic parameters stabilize, and she becomes more comfortable. Her parents are actively involved in her care, report satisfaction with her care, and appreciate the team's dedication to managing her pain, improving her mobility, and obtaining the necessary resources post-discharge.
	She is transferred to a regular inpatient room in preparation for discharge.

was admitted to the PICU. For further information on the nursing care Isabella received related to her pain management, please read the case study details in **Table 3**.

RECOMMENDATIONS FOR THE CRITICAL CARE NURSE

Pediatric pain management in critical care settings requires a specialized approach to ensure the well-being and comfort of young patients. Following are some recommendations for critical care nurses when managing pediatric pain.

Assessment and Monitoring

Regularly assess the child's pain using age-appropriate organization-approved pain assessment tools, considering their developmental stage and communication ability. In addition to the pain assessment tool, use a combination of self-report, behavioral, and physiologic indicators to evaluate pain severity. Physiologic indicators include monitoring vital signs, including heart rate, respiratory rate, blood pressure, and oxygen saturation, as changes in these parameters can indicate pain or distress.

Family-Centered Care

Critical care nurses recognize that pain experiences vary among pediatric patients, so they must tailor pain management strategies to each child's unique needs. When determining pain management approaches, one should consider the child's medical history, surgical procedures, SDOH, and cultural background. Involve the child's family in the decision-making process regarding pain management strategies. Respect cultural beliefs and practices related to pain and pain management.

Non-pharmacologic Treatments

Incorporate non-pharmacologic interventions such as distraction, guided imagery, music therapy, and comfort measures to help alleviate pain and anxiety. The nurse or a child life specialist should engage in therapeutic play and activities that create positive experiences and promote relaxation.

Pharmacologic Interventions

Administer analgesic medications as prescribed, verifying the appropriate doses and routes based on the child's age, weight, and medical condition. Use multimodal analgesia when possible, combining different classes of pain medications for synergistic effects and reduced reliance on opioids. Monitor for potential side effects of medications, including respiratory depression, nausea, constipation, and cognitive dysfunction.

Pain Prevention

Implement pain management strategies and routine assessment proactively to prevent pain from occurring or escalating. Administer pre-emptive analgesia or non-pharmaceutical therapies before painful procedures or activities, such as wound care or turning. Continuously reassess the child's pain level and response to interventions, adjusting the pain management plan as needed. Be alert to changes in the child's condition that might impact pain perception or treatment effectiveness.

Communication and Education

Establish effective communication with the child and their parents or caregivers, explaining the pain management plan and addressing concerns. Educate parents on recognizing signs of pain in their child and encourage their active involvement in pain assessment and management.

Collaboration

To ensure comprehensive care, collaborate with a multidisciplinary team, including physicians, child life specialists, psychologists, respiratory therapists, and pain management experts. Share observations and insights with team members to collectively optimize pain management strategies.

Documentation

Document pain assessments, interventions, and outcomes accurately and comprehensively in the patient's medical record. Ensure clear communication of pain management details during shift handoffs to maintain continuity of care.

Advocate for the Child

Serve as an advocate for the child's pain management needs, prioritizing their comfort and well-being.

Effective pediatric pain management requires sensitivity, empathy, and ongoing assessment. By employing a holistic and tailored approach, critical care nurses can contribute significantly to the recovery and overall experience of pediatric patients in their care.

SUMMARY

In conclusion, the landscape of pediatric pain management is evolving rapidly, emphasizing tailored pharmacologic and non-pharmacologic interventions and sophisticated pain assessment tools. Critical care nurses must stay up to date through nurse education and training in pediatric pain management while recognizing barriers. Integrating these approaches paves the way for more effective and individualized care for young patients, promoting their comfort, well-being, and improved quality of life.

CLINICS CARE POINTS

- Pediatric pain management for critical care nurses is complex. It includes thorough assessment and monitoring of pain, multimodal pain management, multidisciplinary team collaboration, family involvement, prevention of escalation, and documentation.

- Nurses must take a holistic approach to pediatric pain management by considering SDOH and evaluating parents and their own perceptions, beliefs, and biases that can hinder assessing and managing children's pain.

- Nurses face barriers in pediatric pain management due to developmental factors, communication challenges, workload issues, education, and system deficits.

- Education and training are necessary to keep critical care nurses abreast of current and future acute care assessment skills and management of pediatric pain.

DISCLOSURE

The authors have nothing to disclose.

REFERENCES

1. Ismail A. The challenges of providing effective pain management for children in the pediatric intensive care unit. Pain Manag Nurs 2016;17(6):372–83.
2. Sabeti F, Mohammadpour M, Pouraboli B, et al. Health care providers' experiences of the non-pharmacological pain and anxiety management and its barriers in the pediatric intensive care units. J Pediatr Nurs 2021;60:e110–6.
3. Garcia Guerra G, Joffe AR, Sheppard C, et al. Music use for sedation in critically ill children (MUSiCC trial): a pilot randomized controlled trial. J Intensive Care 2021;9(1):7.
4. Gartley CE. Pediatric pain management. Am Nurse. 2021. Available at: https://www.myamericannurse.com/pediatric-pain-management-individualized-approach/. [Accessed 17 August 2023].
5. Khalil NS. Critical care nurses' use of non-pharmacological pain management methods in Egypt. Appl Nurs Res 2018;44:33–8.

6. Hartley S, Redmond T, Berry K. Therapeutic relationships within child and adolescent mental health inpatient services: a qualitative exploration of the experiences of young people, family members and nursing staff. PLoS One 2022;17(1):e0262070.

7. Ismail A, Forgeron P, Polomeno V, et al. Pain management interventions in the paediatric intensive care Unit: a scoping review. Intensive Crit Care Nurs 2019;54:96–105.

8. Ouyang F, Zheng L, Jiao P. Artificial intelligence in online higher education: a systematic review of empirical research from 2011 to 2020. Educ Inf Technol 2022; 27(6):7893–925.

9. Wren AA, Ross AC, D'Souza G, et al. Multidisciplinary pain management for pediatric patients with acute and chronic pain: a foundational treatment approach when prescribing opioids. Children 2019;6(2):33.

10. Goyal MK, Johnson TJ, Chamberlain JM, et al. Racial and ethnic differences in emergency Department pain management of children with fractures. Pediatrics 2020;145(5):e20193370.

11. Apaydın Cırık V, Çiftçioğlu Ş, Efe E. Knowledge, Practice and beliefs of pediatric nurses about pain. J Pediatr Res 2019;6(3):220–7.

12. Liu YM, Lin GL, Chao KY, et al. Comparison of the effectiveness of teaching strategies for a pediatric pain management program for undergraduate nursing students: a quantitative evaluation using an objective structured clinical examination. Nurse Educ Pract 2020;43:102707.

13. Smeland AH, Twycross A, Lundeberg S, et al. Educational intervention to strengthen pediatric postoperative pain m,nagement: a cluster randomized trial. Pain Manag Nurs 2022;23(4):430–42.

14. Chen YC, Peng NH, Chen CH, et al. Effectiveness of pain and symptom management training for paediatric clinicians. J Res Nurs 2017;22(5):405–15.

15. Aziznejadroshan P, Alhani F, Mohammadi E. Experience of nurses about barriers to pain management in pediatric units: a qualitative study. J Nurs Midwifery Sci 2017;4(3):89.

16. Uwimana P, Mukamana D, Adejumo O, et al. Facilitation of nursing students' competency acquisition for paediatric pain management in low- and middle-income countries: a scoping review. Res J Health Sci 2021;9(1):82–99.

17. Ortiz MI, Ponce-Monter HA, Rangel-Flores E, et al. Nurses' and nursing students' knowledge and attitudes regarding pediatric pain. Nurs Res Pract 2015;2015:1–8.

18. Aydın B, Bektaş M. Pediatric pain management knowledge scale for nursing students: assessment of the psychometric properties. J Pediatr Res 2021;8(1):82–92.

19. Trottier ED, Ali S, Doré-Bergeron MJ, et al. Best practices in pain assessment and management for children. Paediatr Child Health 2022;27(7):429–37.

20. ANA Position Statement: the ethical responsibility to manage pain and the suffering it causes. OJIN Online J Issues Nurs 2018;24(1). https://doi.org/10. 3912/OJIN.Vol24No01PoSCol01.

21. Wuni A, Salia SM, Mohammed IM, et al. Evaluating knowledge, practices, and barriers of paediatric pain management among nurses in a tertiary health facility in the northern region of Ghana: a descriptive cross-sectional study. Pain Res Manag 2020;2020:1–11.

22. Thornton M, Persaud S. Preparing Today's Nurses: social determinants of health and nursing education. OJIN Online J Issues Nurs 2018;23(3). https://doi.org/10. 3912/OJIN.Vol23No03Man05.

23. Wakefield EO, Kissi A, Mulchan SS, et al. Pain-related stigma as a social determinant of health in diverse pediatric pain populations. Front Pain Res 2022;3:1020287.

24. LaFond CM, Van Hulle Vincent C, Corte C, et al. PICU Nurses' Pain assessments and intervention choices for virtual human and written vignettes. J Pediatr Nurs 2015;30(4):580–90.

25. Treiman-Kiveste A, Pölkki T, Kalda R, et al. Nurses' perceptions of infants' procedural pain assessment and alleviation with non-pharmacological methods in Estonia. J Pediatr Nurs 2022;62:e156–63.

26. Taam B, Lim F. Best Practices in Pediatric oncology pain management. Am J Nurs 2023;123(5):52–8.

27. Capolingua M, Gill FJ. Neonatal nurses' self-reported practices, knowledge and attitudes toward premature infant pain assessment and management. J Neonatal Nurs 2018;24(4):218–24.

28. Bennett M. Pain assessment and management in paediatric intensive care: Part 1. Paediatr Care 2001;13(5):26–8.

29. Brand K, Al-Rais A. Pain assessment in children. Anaesth Intensive Care Med 2019;20(6):314–7.

30. Social determinants of health. Available at: https://www.who.int/health-topics/social-determinants-of-health. [Accessed 19 January 2024].

31. Sokol R, Austin A, Chandler C, et al. Screening children for social determinants of health: a systematic review. Pediatrics 2019;144(4):e20191622.

32. Andrist E, Riley CL, Brokamp C, et al. Neighborhood poverty and pediatric intensive care use. Pediatrics 2019;144(6):e20190748.

33. Akande M, Paquette ET, Magee P, et al. Screening for cocial determinants of health in the pediatric intensive care unit. Crit Care Clin 2023;39(2):341–55.

34. Perez NP, Ahmad H, Alemayehu H, et al. The impact of social determinants of health on the overall wellbeing of children: a review for the pediatric surgeon. J Pediatr Surg 2022;57(4):587–97.

35. Xiao Y, Mann JJ, Chow JCC, et al. Patterns of social determinants of health and child mental health, cognition, and physical health. JAMA Pediatr 2023;177(12):1294.

36. Brown L, França UL, McManus ML. Neighborhood poverty and distance to pediatric hospital care. Acad Pediatr 2023;23(6):1276–81.

37. Moen M, Storr C, German D, et al. A review of tools to screen for social determinants of health in the United States: a practice brief. Popul Health Manag 2020;23(6):422–9.

38. Screening tool finder. Available at: https://www.aap.org/en/patient-care/screening-technical-assistance-and-resource-center/screening-tool-finder/. [Accessed 19 January 2024].

39. Ward M, Ellis PL. Pediatrics: Addressing social determinants of health and adverse childhood Experiences. The Doctors Company. ://www.thedoctors.com/articles/pediatrics- addressing- social-determinants-of-health-and-adverse-childhood-experiences/.

40. Dongara AR, Nimbalkar SM, Phatak AG, et al. An educational intervention to improve nurses' understanding of pain in children in western India. Pain Manag Nurs 2017;18(1):24–32.

41. Palomaa AK, Hakala M, Pölkki T. Parents' perceptions of their child's pain assessment in hospital care: a cross-sectional study. J Pediatr Nurs 2023;71:79–87.

42. Kammerer E, Eszczuk J, Caldwell K, et al. A qualitative study of the pain experiences of children and their parents at a Canadian children's hospital. Children 2022;9(12):1796.

43. AlReshidi N, Long T, Darvill A. A systematic review of the impact of educational programs on factors that affect nurses' post-operative pain management for children. Compr Child Adolesc Nurs 2018;41(1):9–24.

44. Vagnoli L, Mammucari M, Graziani D, et al. Doctors and nurses' knowledge and attitudes towards pediatric pain management: an exploratory survey in a children's hospital. J Pain Palliat Care Pharmacother 2019;33(3–4):107–19.

45. Alghadeer SM, Wajid S, Babelghaith SD, et al. Assessment of Saudi mothers' attitudes towards their children's pain and its management. Int J Environ Res Public Health 2021;18(1):348.

46. Yu KE, Kim JS. Pediatric Postoperative Pain management in Korea: parental attitudes toward pain and analgesics, self-efficacy, and pain management. J Pediatr Nurs 2021;58:e28–36.

47. Shrestha-Ranjit J, Ranjitkar UD, Water T, et al. Nurses' knowledge and attitudes regarding children's pain assessment and management in Nepal. J Child Health Care 2023. https://doi.org/10.1177/13674935231195133. 13674935231195133.

48. Raphael JL, Oyeku SO. Implicit bias in pediatrics: an emerging focus in health equity research. Pediatrics 2020;145(5):e20200512.

49. Davis S, O'Brien AM. Fast fact about diversity, equity, and inclusion in nursing. Building competencies for an antiracism practice. New York, NY: Springer Publishing; 2023.

50. Sabin JA, Greenwald AG. The influence of implicit bias on treatment recommendations for 4 common pediatric conditions: pain, urinary tract infection, attention deficit hyperactivity disorder, and asthma. Am J Public Health 2012;102(5):988–95.

51. Groenewald CB, Rabbitts JA, Hansen EE, et al. Racial differences in opioid prescribing for children in the United States. Pain 2018;159(10):2050–7.

52. Earp BD, Monrad JT, LaFrance M, et al. Featured article: gender bias in pediatric pain assessment. J Pediatr Psychol 2019;44(4):403–14.

53. Cohen LL, Cobb J, Martin SR. Gender biases in adult ratings of pediatric pain. Child Health Care 2014;43(2):87–95.

54. Miller MM, Williams AE, Zapolski TCB, et al. Assessment and treatment recommendations for pediatric pain: the influence of patient race, patient gender, and provider pain-related attitudes. J Pain 2020;21(1–2):225–37.

55. Zhang L, Losin EAR, Ashar YK, et al. Gender biases in estimation of others' pain. J Pain 2021;22(9):1048–59.

56. Guedj R, Marini M, Kossowsky J, et al. Racial and ethnic disparities in pain management of children with limb fractures or suspected appendicitis: a retrospective cross-sectional study. Front Pediatr 2021;9:652854.

57. Eccleston C, Fisher E, Howard RF, et al. Delivering transformative action in paediatric pain: a Lancet child & adolescent health Commission. Lancet Child Adolesc Health 2021;5(1):47–87.

58. O'Neal K, Olds D. Differences in Pediatric pain management by unit types: pediatric pain management. J Nurs Scholarsh 2016;48(4):378–86.

59. Rosen DM, Alcock MM, Palmer GM. Opioids for acute pain management in children. Anaesth Intensive Care 2022;50(1–2):81–94.

60. Grogan S, Preuss CV. Pharmacokinetics. In: StatPearls. Treasure island (FL): StatPearls Publishing. 2023. Available at: http://www.ncbi.nlm.nih.gov/books/NBK557744/. [Accessed 23 August 2023].

61. Kia Z, Allahbakhshian M, Ilkhani M, et al. Nurses' use of non-pharmacological pain management methods in intensive care units: a descriptive cross-sectional study. Complement Ther Med 2021;58:102705.

62. Hypnosis for postoperative pain management of Thoracoscopic... : J of Pediatr Surg Nurs. Available at: https://journals.lww.com/journalofpediatricsurgicalnursing/abstract/2015/04000/hypnosis_for_postoperative_pain_management_of.6.aspx. [Accessed 23 August 2023].

63. Matula ST, Irving SY, Deatrick JA, et al. The perceptions and practices of parents and children on acute pain management among hospitalized children in two Botswana referral hospitals. J Pediatr Nurs 2022;65:e35–42.

Longitudinal Pain Management Claims in Maryland: Implications

George A. Zangaro, PhD, RN[a],*, William O. Howie, CRNA, DNP[b],
Patricia C. McMullen, PhD, JD, CRNP[c],
Benjamin A. Fujita-Howie, MD, MPH[d]

KEYWORDS

- Pain management • Claims • Malpractice • Patient safety

KEY POINTS

- Analysis of closed pain-related claims revealed a need for improved patient education, outcomes, quality, and safety.
- Contemporary research indicates that practicing critical event simulation training has the potential for reducing serious adverse outcomes.
- Results indicated that the number of pain-related malpractice claims in Maryland has increased from 1996 to 2023, which is consistent with national trends.
- Proactive measures can be implemented by the health care industry to reduce legal liability while also improving the quality and safety of patient care.

INTRODUCTION

Millions of Americans experience persistent pain and require treatment by providers who specialize in pain management. According to Rikard and colleagues,[1] in 2021 an estimated 51.6 million (20.9%) US adults experienced chronic pain. Anesthesiologists are among the primary providers of pain management and utilize medications and interventional approaches in conjunction with physical therapists and behavioral health experts to control pain, with other types of providers now offering such services as well. Medical malpractice claims associated with pain management have increased over the last several decades.

[a] American Association of Colleges of Nursing, 655 K Street Northwest, Washington, DC 20001, USA; [b] R. Adams Cowley Shock Trauma Center, 22 S. Greene St, Baltimore, MD 20121, USA; [c] Conway School of Nursing, The Catholic University of America, 620 Michigan Avenue, NE, Washington DC 20064, USA; [d] Pain Medicine Department, Icahan School of Medicine & Mt Sinai Medical Center, 100 5th Ave New York, NY 10011, USA
* Corresponding author. American Association of Colleges of Nursing, 655 K Street, NW Suite 750, Washington, DC 20001.
E-mail address: gzangaro@aacnnursing.org

Crit Care Nurs Clin N Am 36 (2024) 495–504
https://doi.org/10.1016/j.cnc.2024.04.005
0899-5885/24/© 2024 Elsevier Inc. All rights reserved.

The purpose of this study was to conduct a longitudinal review of pain management claims filed in the state of Maryland. The analysis of closed claims promotes open interprofessional discussions among peers and organizations to improve pain management and patient safety and promote positive patient outcomes.

METHODS

As was noted in prior publications, a unique source of information in Maryland is available through the Health Care Alternative Dispute Resolution Office.[2,3] Under Maryland law, all legal claims against a health care provider that originate in Maryland must initially be submitted to this office.[3] In some instances, involved parties may agree to arbitrate a matter in lieu of a formal trial. More often, a claimant, whether plaintiff (person filing the claim) or defendant (individual or health care agency alleged to have caused the injury), may waive arbitration and move forward to a formal trial once they have filed a certificate of merit by a qualified medical expert with the director of the Health Claims Arbitration Office.[4] Once waiver of arbitration has occurred, the relevant parties proceed either to drop the claim and settle the matter or to have the case tried in the County Circuit Court in the county where the alleged malpractice occurred because the Circuit Courts have jurisdiction over claims in excess of US$30,000.[5] Most of these cases are either settled prior to or during trial and such settlements are typically conditioned on the plaintiff's agreement not to disclose the amount of the settlement. As such, the settlement amount is unknown in the majority of cases. Older data indicate that in 2003 there were 688 cases filed, and only 6 cases were arbitrated, with the remainder withdrawn, settled, or tried.[6]

Claims are publicly accessible and do not require institutional review board approval to access claims information. One member from the research team traveled to the Health Care Alternative Dispute Resolution Office and manually accessed all claims that used the terms anesthesia, anesthetic, CRNA (certified registered nurse anesthetist), and anesthesiologist. From these data, claims involving pain procedures were selected and analyzed for pain-specific malpractice analysis. Two of the team members independently reviewed these records and obtained specific data points; any disagreements were resolved by consensus.

Statistical Analysis

The current secondary data analysis analyzed closed-malpractice claims focusing on pain that were filed with the Maryland Health Claims Arbitration Office between 1996 and 2023. Specifically, this study analyzed (1) demographics of the sample, (2) venue where claim occurred, (3) facility type, (4) provider type, (5) causes of action, and (6) patient outcomes. Descriptive statistics were used to describe the sample and clinical outcome variables. The years the claims were filed were divided into 3 categories for analysis: (1) 1996 to 2004, (2) 2005 to 2013, and (3) 2014 to 2023. The cause of action variable was a multiple response option and was analyzed using a multiple response analysis. This type of analysis permits the combing of the set of responses and the collective analysis of those responses. Each response option was coded separately with the value of 1 if the cause occurred and 0 if the cause did not occur. The analysis was conducted using Statistical Package for the Social Sciences (SPSS) version 27.

RESULTS

The pain-related claims included in this analysis occurred between 1996 and 2023. **Table 1** provides a summary of characteristics of the pain-related claims included in our sample. There was a total of 17,929 claims filed in the state of Maryland from

Table 1 Characteristics of filed claims		
Variables	**Total Claims (N = 94)**	
	Mean	*SD*
Age (n = 55)	51.7	16.9
	n	*%*
Gender (n = 94)		
Male	34	36.2
Female	60	63.8
Year claim filed (n = 94)		
1996–2004	13	13.8
2005–2013	20	21.3
2014–2023	61	64.9
Facility type (n = 93)		
Teaching hospital	11	11.8
Community hospital	15	16.1
Out-patient surgery center	55	59.2
Provider's office	11	11.8
Urgent care	1	1.1
Provider type (n = 94)		
Anesthesiologist (MDA)	89	94.7
MDA/CRNA	3	3.2
MDA/Resident	1	1.1
CRNA	1	1.1
American Society of Anesthesiologists (ASA) Criteria (n = 94)		
ASA I: Normal	1	1.1
ASA II: Mild systemic disease	70	74.5
ASA III: Severe systemic disease	23	24.5
County where event occurred (n = 91)		
Baltimore	46	50.5
Baltimore city	15	16.5
Prince Georges	4	4.4
Montgomery	6	6.6
Anne Arundel	3	3.3
Carroll	1	1.1
Frederick	2	2.2
Charles	2	2.2
Howard	1	1.1
Washington	4	4.4
Kent	1	1.1
Prince Frederick	1	1.1
Harford	5	5.5

Note: Percentages represent the valid percent based on number of respondents and may not total to 100.0 due to rounding.

1996 to 2023 and of those 94 (0.52%) were pain-related claims. Age is not required to be reported in any filed claim. As a result, the patient age was reported in 55 of the 94 cases, with an average age of 51.7 years. Most patients, 63.8%, were female. Over half of the cases (n = 61, 64.9%) occurred between 2014 and 2023. Roughly 95% (n = 89) of the claims were filed against physicians, with 27% (n = 24) of those claims being filed against one physician. Twenty of the 24 claims against this one physician occurred at one facility, 2 occurred at another facility, and 2 in a surgical center. Of the 24 claims filed against the same physician, 5 of the 24 resulted in patient deaths; 11 patients reported pain, suffering, and emotional distress; 6 patients with back spinal cord injury; 1 patient with brain damage; and 1 patient with neck and spine injury.

In addition, these claims all occurred between 2014 and 2023. Out-patient surgery centers experienced the largest percentage of claims (59.2%), which is not surprising given that most pain procedures have moved out of the hospital setting. There were 13 different counties in Maryland where an incident resulted in a claim. Of these 13 counties, 67% of these events occurred in Baltimore County (50.5%) and Baltimore City (16.5%), 2 of the largest venues in Maryland.

Table 2 depicts the pain-related legal causes of action or critical events that led to the alleged adverse patient outcomes. The first percentage in the table represents the percentage of the total number of causes of action (N = 274) and the second percentage is based on the total number of claims (N = 94). While there are 94 claims in the file, there were a total of 274 causes of action because each claim may have had multiple causes of action associated with it. The majority of claims reported inappropriate pain service management (n = 88; 93.6%); inadequate informed consent (n = 55; 58.5%); inappropriate medication (n = 48; 51.1%); and inappropriate charting (n = 45; 16.4%) as the most frequent causes of action. There were several other causes of action reported, but they each occurred in less than 10% of the claims.

As reflected in **Table 3**, the top 3 patient outcomes that were reported included pain, suffering, and emotional distress (n = 33; 35.1%), back spinal cord injury (n = 22; 23.4%), and death (n = 22; 23.4%). There were 10 claims that included brain damage (9.6%) as a patient outcome. Each of the remaining patient outcomes accounted for less than 5% of the claims.

Table 2 Causes of action			
Causes of Action	n	% of Causes (N = 274)	% of Claims (N = 94)
Inappropriate pain service management	88	32.1	93.6
Inadequate informed consent	55	20.1	58.5
Inappropriate medication	48	17.5	51.1
Inappropriate charting	45	16.4	47.9
Failure to respond to postoperative changes	9	3.3	9.6
Failure to properly administer anesthesia	6	2.2	6.4
Inappropriate medication dosage	5	1.8	5.3
Improper epidural	5	1.8	5.3
Inadequate preoperative	4	1.5	4.3
Failure to monitor	4	1.5	4.3
Failure to secure airway/ventilate/aspirate	2	0.7	2.1
Failure to respond to intraoperative changes	2	0.7	2.1
Fall	1	0.4	1.1

Table 3 Patient outcomes		
Patient Outcome	N = 94	%
Pain, suffering, and emotional distress	33	35.1
Death	22	23.4
Back spinal cord injury	22	23.4
Brain damage	10	10.6
Neck spine injury	3	3.2
Nerve damage	1	1.1
Severe drug reaction	1	1.1
Broken bones	1	1.1
Narcotic withdrawal leading to myocardial infarction	1	1.1

Note: Percentages are valid percentages and may not total to 100.0 due to rounding.

DISCUSSION AND IMPLICATIONS

The current research study analyzed closed claims malpractice data for pain-related procedures over a 27 year period. At commencement of the research study, our purpose was to garner salient factors implicated in pain-related malpractice claims and better understand resulting patient adverse outcomes. By uncovering the most common causes for these adverse outcomes, investigators aimed to propose strategies to reduce the risk of patient harm and subsequent litigation following pain procedures, while improving quality of care. The discussion that follows will underscore key takeaways from our study and offer potential strategies in ameliorating adverse patient outcomes and improving the quality of pain-related care.

Results from the current study indicate that the number of pain-related malpractice claims in Maryland increased from 1996 to 2023 (1996–2004: 13; 2005–2013: 20; 2014–2023: 61). In the state of Maryland during these same time periods, pain-related claims accounted for 0.21% (1996–2004; n = 6076), 0.34% (2005–2013; n = 5914), and 1.03% (2014–2023; n = 5939) of the total number of malpractice claims. These trends are consistent with national trends published using the National Practitioner Database. Additionally, study by Pollak and colleagues, who analyzed 5709 total malpractice claims, reported in the National Practitioner Database, indicated that nationally the number of pain medicine-related claims increased from 3% between 1980 and 2012 up to 18% between 2000 and 2012 (total number of pain-related malpractice claims during study period: 1037).[7] Similarly, as seen in our study, data highlighted by the Pollak research team underscores an increase in the percentage of claims that resulted in death or permanent disability over the analyzed 32 year period. While it is unclear the exact reason for this increase in claims involving death and permanent disability, possible reasons may include increased volume (ie, total patient numerator) of pain procedures over the study period; an increase in the number and type of advanced interventional pain procedures requiring monitored anesthesia or general anesthesia at ambulatory surgery centers; greater procedural complexity, or greater production pressure resulting from increased patient volume. Furthermore, nearly a quarter of the reported deaths during the study period occurred at the hands of a single provider, thus underscoring possible skewing of the data toward higher extremes as a result of a single outlier provider.

It should be mentioned that some of the cases in our data set may have been associated with the New England Compounding Center. Briefly, in 2012, 753 patients in 20 states were diagnosed with fungal meningitis following receipt of epidural injections of contaminated preservative-free methylprednisolone acetate that had been manufactured by the New England Compounding Center, resulting in 100 patient deaths in 9 states. As of 2018, 11 former owners, executives and employees have been convicted of federal criminal charges associated with these injuries and deaths.[8] Unfortunately, production and distribution of contaminated neuraxial pain medications have persisted. Specifically, 2 surgical centers in Matamoros Tamaulipas, Mexico were closed in 2023 when it was determined that of 547 procedures, 20 patients presented with symptoms of meningitis following neuraxial anesthetic procedures at the centers. Two hundred thirty-seven of these patients were from the United States.[9]

Much of the research on adverse patient outcomes and legal liability found that typically physician providers had the most claims, likely because originally most pain management was under the province of physician providers. However, of late, there has been an increasing frequency of pain-related care delivered by either those who are not physicians or who are physicians but are not anesthesiologists (pain-boarded neurologists, physiatrists, orthopedists, nurse practitioners, and CRNAs), warranting future research on adverse patient outcomes that includes such providers.[10–12] Consequently, although much of the research is physician-focused, attention to these findings is relevant to nonphysicians handling pain management cases as well.

Unfortunately, as indicated in the present study, adverse outcomes in the pain-related claims are often severe and included death, brain damage, and back and spinal cord sequelae. In a subsequent review, Studdert noted physicians often claim that medicolegal events strike randomly and arbitrarily.[13] However, research indicates that there are well-documented factors, both on the provider side (eg, communication skills and male gender) and the patient side (eg, serious adverse outcomes of care) associated with the adverse patient outcomes.[14,15]

More evidence is needed to determine what works to restore medicolegal event–prone providers to safe practice, or, when necessary, to shepherd them away from patient care.[13] Future patient safety initiatives offer potential solutions and will likely include a multipronged approach to ensure adequate patient-informed consent, standardized timeout procedures to ensure the correct procedure and correct laterality for the correct patient, preprocedural checklists to address potential patient safety risk factors, and harm mitigation contingencies when adverse outcomes do arise. Contemporary research does indicate that practicing critical event simulation training has the potential for reducing serious adverse outcomes.[16] Furthermore, placing cognitive aids, such as emergency management algorithms that reflect proper procedures in the event of an adverse event in areas where these procedures are performed, may ameliorate negative patient sequelae.[17]

Two older research studies support the findings of the present analysis. Specifically, in a 2016 study of claims placed in the National Practitioner Data Bank (NPDB) from 2005 to 2014, Studdert and colleagues employed multivariable recurrent-event survival analysis to identify characteristics of physicians who had a higher risk for recurrent claims. Additionally, they quantified longitudinal risk levels across all health care specialties.[18] Of the 66,426 paid claims in the NPDB, 32% were attributable to approximately 1% of all physicians. An adjusted analysis indicated that the risk of additional claims increased with the number of previously paid claims. Certain specialties had higher risk of recurrence, including neurosurgery, orthopedic surgery, general surgery, and plastic surgery, respectively.[18,19] Psychiatrists and pediatricians had the lowest risk of recurrence. In terms of demographics, male individuals, nonresident physicians, and Medical Doctors (MDs) (vs Doctor of Osteopathic Medicine [DOs]) had a lower frequency of increased claims. Anesthesiologists had the third lowest number of claims.

Consistent with the findings of Studdert, our research determined that of the total 94 claims, one provider was named in 24 of the claims (27%) and one center accounted for 24.4% of the claims. This highlights the importance of proactive measures including early identification of at-risk providers and centers, adherence to evidenced-based practice guidelines, continuous quality improvement activities, remediation, increased supervision, board certification in interventional pain, and withdrawal of credentials when warranted.[20,21] We contend that like the airline industry, the health care industry can implement proactive measures to reduce legal liability while also improving the quality of patient care. As reflected in this study, as well as a prior study we authored,[2] patient safety policies and practices should be designed by practitioners on the frontlines of care to promote a health care system that will learn from successes and failures with the goal of improving patient outcomes and efficient overall function.

Given the subjective nature of pain, it is recommended that practitioners gather information on the psychological and mental health of the patient. There should be a history of prior use of pain medications (amount, frequency, and type) including an explanation as to why the pain medication was being used. Reporting and documenting any history of substance abuse is critical, as well as ensuring appropriate pain management protocols are used. Additionally, utilization of nonpharmacologic therapies, such as transcutaneous electrical nerve stimulation, massage therapy, ultrasound therapy, hypnosis, mindfulness, and cognitive behavioral therapy, has proven helpful in the management of chronic pain and some patients may report they are using or are willing to try such therapies.[22]

Despite the fact that patient safety in anesthesia practice has steadily improved over the last few decades, patient safety policies should ideally support a "learning health system" approach to safety, in which measurement on the front lines of care creates evidence for improvement. The evidence should be used in an ongoing way to develop interventions that are incorporated into practice, rather than for punitive purposes.

Investigators argue that an understanding of the underlying causes implicated in a malpractice claim is essential in mitigating the risk of a future claim.[23] The 4 most salient causes of action in our study were inappropriate pain service management (32.1%), inadequate informed consent (20.1%), inappropriate medication (17.5%), and inappropriate charting (16.4%). Consequently, a thorough review of the pain patient's diagnosis, a discussion of potential treatment options and associated risks and benefits of said options, and attention to patient's underlying medical history (medical comorbidities, allergies, current medications, and prior pain treatment history), physical examination findings, and relevant laboratory and test findings (ie, MRI, computed tomography, radiographs, and electromyography if indicated) is warranted. Additionally, proposed assessment and management should be thoroughly outlined and discussed with the patient and the above-mentioned informed consent process should be undertaken with attention to documentation of discussed risks and benefits associated with planned procedures. Adherence to these points can aid clinicians in increased levels of patient satisfaction, and risk mitigation. Thorough documentation of the informed consent process can be invaluable should litigation arise.

LIMITATIONS

Several limitations exist based on the design of this study. First, retrospective closed claims data limitations have been previously documented and include selection bias, outcome bias, the nonrandomized nature of retrospectively collected data, and limitations in claims data based on insurance collections during the course of the malpractice claims resolution.[19] Additionally, although our data would suggest that the percentage in claims increased during the study period, the denominator of total number of procedures performed or patients seen is unknown. Lastly, as mentioned in the introduction to this study, most settlements that occur prior to or during a trial are contingent on sealing the actual financial award to be paid by the defendant. As such, the mean and range settlement sum cannot be determined from the analyzed pain-related malpractice claims.

SUMMARY

With millions of Americans experiencing both acute and chronic pain, pain management providers are a vital part of the health care team. There is a lot to be learned from past experiences, identified in these closed pain management claims, specifically on how to improve patient education, quality, and safety. Unfortunately, there is still no national repository for all medical errors. Such data could be used to devise strategies that support continuous quality improvement, minimize preventable adverse events, and reduce both human and economic costs.

CLINICS CARE POINTS

- Providers have access to the National Practitioner Data Bank, a federal source that allows them to determine specific areas of practice that place them at particular risk. They can then tailor their quality improvement initiatives based on specific areas of concern.

- With the increase in care that is delivered in outpatient settings, providers should have "drills" or other ways to ensure those delivering care in outpatient settings are able to respond appropriately to critical situations that have rare occurrence rates.

- A longitudinal review of existing data from the National Practitioner Data Bank, as well as from evidence-based research studies, indicates that a disproportionate number of adverse events are associated with a small number of providers. Those providers who are identified as having higher numbers of adverse events should receive additional education and training and some will require more stringent monitoring.

DISCLOSURE

The authors have nothing to disclose. The views, analyses, and conclusions expressed in this article are those of the authors and do not necessarily reflect the official policy or positions of the American Association of Colleges of Nursing.

REFERENCES

1. Rikard SM, Strahan AE, Schmit KM, et al. Chronic pain among adults — United States, 2019–2021. MMWR Morb Mortal Wkly Rep 2023;72:379–85.
2. Howie WO, Zangaro G, Howie BA, et al. Anesthesia-related malpractice claims in Maryland 1994-2017. AANA J (Am Assoc Nurse Anesth) 2022;90(6):455–61.
3. MD.ANN.CODE, Art 48A Secs. 548-556 (1979). Chapter 235, Acts of 1976.
4. McAlister JK, Scanlon AL. Health claims arbitration in Maryland: the experiment has failed. Univ Baltim Law Rev 1985;14(3):481–521.
5. Judiciary MD. Div. Of government relations and public affairs. Maryland's judicial system. Available at: https://www.courts.state.md.us/sites/default/files/import/publications/pdfs/mdjudicialsystem.pdf. [Accessed 10 January 2024].

6. Schulte F, Salganik MW. Malpractice arbitration in MD called a failure. Baltimore Sun; 2004. Available at: https://www.baltimoresun.com/news/bs-xpm-2004-11-27-0411270354-story.html. [Accessed 10 January 2024].

7. Pollak KA, Stephens LS, Posner KL, et al. Trends in pain medicine liability. Anesthesiology 2015;123(5):1133–41.

8. U.S. Food & Drug Administration. Owner and four former employees of New England Compounding Center convicted following trial. 2018. Available at: https://www.fda.gov/inspections-compliance-enforcement-and-criminal-investigations/press-releases/december-13-2018-owner-and-four-former-employees-new-en gland-compounding-center-convicted-following. [Accessed 10 January 2024].

9. World Health Organization. Outbreak of suspected fungal meningitis associated with surgical procedures performed under spinal anesthesia -The United States of American & Mexico. 2023. Available at: https://www.who.int/emergencies/disease-outbreak-news/item/2023-DON470. [Accessed 11 January 2024].

10. American Society of Interventional Pain Physicians. About us. 2024. Available at: https://asipp.org/duplicated-about-asipp-87/. [Accessed 14 January 2024].

11. American Association of Nurse Practitioners. Pain management specialty practice group. 2024. Pain management specialty practice group (aanp.org). Available at: https://www.aanp.org/membership/aanp-communities/pain-management-spg. Accessed January 16, 2024.

12. American Association of Nurse Anesthetists. Clinical pain management. 2024. Clinical pain management - AANA - American association of nurse anesthesiology. Available at: https://www.aana.com/practice/clinical-practice/clinical-practice-resources/clinical-pain-management/. Accessed January 18, 2024.

13. Studdert D. Doctors with multiple malpractice claims, disciplinary actions, and complaints: what do we know?, AHRQ Patient Safety Network. 2017. Doctors With Multiple Malpractice Claims, Disciplinary Actions, and Complaints: What Do We Know? | PSNet (ahrq.gov). Available at: https://psnet.ahrq.gov/perspective/doctors-multiple-malpractice-claims-disciplinary-actions-and-complaints-what-do-we-know. Accessed February 1, 2024.

14. Gharibo C, Drewes AM, Breve F, et al. Iatrogenic side effects of pain therapies. Cureus 2023;15(9):e44583.

15. LoBianco G, Tinnirello A, Papa A, et al. Interventional pain procedures: a narrative review focusing on safety and complications: Part I injections for spinal pain. J Pain Res 2023;16:1637–46.

16. Wahr JA. Safety in the operating room. UptoDate. Updated September 21, 2023. Patient safety in the operating room - UpToDate. Available at: https://psnet.ahrq.gov/issue/operating-room-hazards-and-approaches-improve-patient-safety. Accessed February 2, 2024.

17. Minehart RD. Cognitive aids for perioperative emergencies. UptoDate. Available at: https://www.uptodate.com/contents/cognitive-aids-for-perioperative-emergencies. [Accessed 2 February 2024].

18. Studdert DM, Bismark MM, Mello MM, et al. Prevalence and characteristics of physicians prone to malpractice claims. N Engl J Med 2016;374(4):354–62.

19. Dziadkowiec O, Durbin J, Muralidharan VJ, et al. Improving the quality and design of retrospective clinical outcome studies that utilize electronic health records. HCA Healthc J Med 2020;1(3):131–8.

20. Chang B, Kaye AD, Diaz JH, et al. Interventional procedures outside of the operating room: results from the national anesthesia clinical outcomes registry. J Patient Saf 2018;14(1):9–16.

21. Manchikanti L, Knezevic NN, Navani A, et al. Epidural interventions in the management of chronic spinal pain: American Society of Interventional Pain Physicians (ASIPP) comprehensive evidence-based guidelines. Pain Physician 2021; 24(S1):S27–208.
22. Shi Y, Wu W. Multimodal non-invasive non-pharmacological therapies for chronic pain: mechanisms and progress. BMC Med 2023;21(1):372.
23. Schwendimann R, Blatter C, Dhaini S, et al. The occurrence, types, consequences and preventability of in-hospital adverse events-a scoping review. BMC Health Serv Res 2018;18(1):521.

Using Simulation to Illustrate Pain

Heather S. Cole, PhD, RN, CHSE, CNEn[a],*,
Mahalia G. Barrow, EdD, RN, CNL[a]

KEY WORDS

- Pain • Simulation • Nursing • Education • Training

KEY POINTS

- Around 51.6 million adults are living with chronic pain that has been shown to lead to mental health disorders, substance use, and suicidal ideation.
- Structured education and training in assessment, management, and collaborative pain treatment are needed to prepare health care professionals to care for diverse patient populations.
- Simulation-based learning is an effective educational modality to train health care professionals to provide high-quality care for patients suffering from pain.

INTRODUCTION

The Centers for Disease Control and Prevention report that in 2021, an estimated 51.6 million adults experienced chronic pain.[1] Living with chronic pain has been linked to mental health conditions, dementia, substance use, and suicidal ideation.[1] Higher rates of pain are also linked to an increase in age and those without a college degree.[2] The high incidence of chronic pain poses a challenge for health care educators to ensure that future health care professionals receive training to assess, prevent, and manage chronic pain for a diverse patient population already suffering from other chronic health conditions. Simulation-based learning is an invaluable resource for training and educating in health care and encompasses multiple modalities, including screen-based computer simulations, standardized patients, high-fidelity mannequins, and low-fidelity task trainers; however, little is known about using simulation-based learning to illustrate pain. This review aims to determine the current evidence related to using simulation-based learning for training and teaching the assessment and management of pain in the nursing discipline.

[a] Capstone College of Nursing, The University of Alabama in Tuscaloosa, AL 35401, USA
* Corresponding author. 650 University Boulevard, E Tuscaloosa, AL 35401.
E-mail address: hscole@ua.edu

Crit Care Nurs Clin N Am 36 (2024) 505–515
https://doi.org/10.1016/j.cnc.2024.04.009
0899-5885/24/© 2024 Elsevier Inc. All rights reserved.

BACKGROUND
Simulation-based Learning

Simulation-based learning experiences are structured activities that resemble realistic or possible scenarios used in the educational and practice settings to train learners in a safe environment.[3] These opportunities allow the learner to develop competence and confidence through deliberate practice with immediate feedback on the learner's performance through debriefing.[4–6] Deliberate practice is intentionally repeating a skill or concept until mastery is achieved. The simulation-based learning experience is intended to promote psychological safety in which learners feel included, safe to acquire knowledge, safe to contribute, and safe to make mistakes without consequence.[7,8] The International Nursing Association for Clinical Simulation provides educators with a framework to ensure that simulation-based learning experiences are developed and aligned with best practice standards.[9] The Healthcare Simulation Standards of Best Practice include (1) professional development, (2) pre-briefing, (3) design, (4) facilitation, (5) debriefing, (6) operations, (7) outcomes and objectives, (8) professional integrity, (9) sim-enhanced interprofessional education (IPE), and (10) evaluation of learning and performance.[9]

Current Guidelines for Pain Education in Nursing

The American Association of Colleges of Nursing Essentials

The American Association of Colleges of Nursing (AACN) is an accrediting body for nursing institutions that outlines expectations for multiple levels of nursing curriculum.[10] The new AACN Essentials is a document that outlines a competency-based framework for baccalaureate entry-level nursing education. This document is categorized into domains, competencies, and subcompetencies that organize a framework of purposeful goals for the nursing curriculum.[10] The expectations for nurses are outlined by 10 domains and 45 competencies. The domains expected for the entry-level new graduate nurse include (1) knowledge of nursing practice, (2) person-centered care, (3) population health, (4) nursing scholarship, (5) quality and safety, (6) interprofessional partnerships, (7) system-based practice, (8) informatics and health care technologies, (9) professionalism, and (10) personal, professional, and leadership development (**Fig. 1**).

Furthermore, the AACN Essentials includes 4 spheres of care that are meant to ensure entry-level nursing students are competent to provide care across the lifespan with a diverse patient population.[10] The 4 spheres of care include (1) wellness and

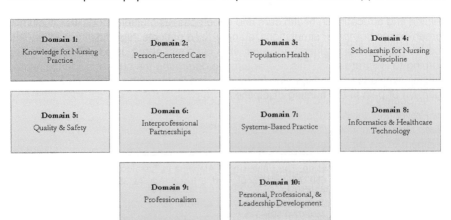

Fig. 1. Core competencies for professional nursing education. (*Data from* AACN, 2021)

disease prevention, (2) chronic disease management, (3) regenerative/restorative care, and (4) hospice and palliative care.[10] While the AACN Essentials does not delineate pain assessment, the outlined domains and spheres of care encompass the skills needed to assess, prevent, and manage pain.[10]

The International Association for the Study of Pain

The International Association for the Study of Pain (IASP) provides curriculum outlines to introduce the knowledge and skills needed to assess and manage pain.[11] Each curriculum is designed for the desired discipline and guides health care educators to embed pain education and training into an existing program of study. The IASP curriculum stresses the fundamental principles of how pain is observed, collaborative efforts for pain management, and applying these principles across the lifespan.[11] The pain curriculum for nursing includes (1) the multidimensional nature of pain, (2) assessment and measurement, (3) pain management, and (4) clinical conditions[11] (**Fig. 2**). When discussing the multidimensional nature of pain, learners are provided the overall anatomy and physiology of pain with an emphasis on biological, psychological, and social factors that impact pain.[11] For assessment and measurement of pain, the curriculum discusses differences across the lifespan, common coping behaviors, patients at risk, and barriers to effective pain management.[11] To discuss pain management, the learner covers pharmacologic and non-pharmacological interventions and the role of the nurse in the interprofessional team.[11] Finally, clinical conditions associated with pain are presented including acute injury, palliative care, end of life, and common chronic conditions.[11] Integrating pain education and training into nursing curriculum ensures that nurses understand their pivotal role and responsibility in assessing and managing pain.

METHODS

To identify primary studies for review, 2 researchers reviewed the literature using the terms *nursing* AND *simulation training* OR *simulation education* OR *simulation learning*

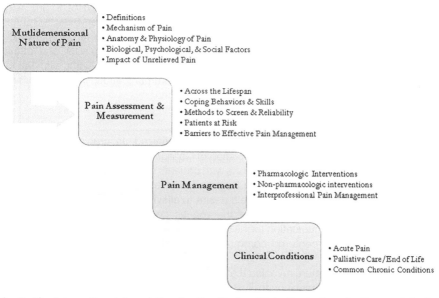

Fig. 2. The International Association for the Study of Pain Curriculum Outline on Pain for Nursing. (*Data from* IASP, 2018)

OR *pain management* OR *pain relief* OR *pain control* OR *pain reduction* AND *critically ill patients* OR *intensive care unit patients* OR *critical care patients*. The databases reviewed through an institutional online library catalog included the Cumulative Index of Nursing and Allied Health Literature Complete, Ovid Lippincott Williams and Wilkins Nursing and Allied Health Professions Premier and Comprehensive Archive Collection, PubMed, and Google Scholar. With the removal of duplicates, the search resulted in 490 combined articles for screening.

The titles and abstracts were screened and narrowed to 103 full-text studies to assess eligibility. Articles under full review were screened for inclusion and exclusion. Inclusion criteria included English, peer-reviewed journal articles from 2019 to 2024 that illustrated pain using simulation-based learning. Exclusion criteria included studies published before 2019 that excluded the nursing discipline and did not utilize simulation as an intervention. Of the 103 articles reviewed, 97 were excluded, with 6 reviewed and categorized into a table of evidence (**Table 1**). The studies were categorized by (1) year of publication, (2) geographic location, (3) theoretic model or framework, (4) research methodology, (5) outcome variables, (6) instrumentation, and (7) quality of evidence using the Grading of Recommendations Assessment and Evaluation (GRADE) guidelines.[12] Articles requiring further consensus on full-text review and inclusion were planned to be reviewed by a third party; however, both researchers reached a consensus on all articles included in this review.

RESULTS

The 6 studies in this review reported outcomes for 1042 participants, including students (n = 847) and practicing nurses (n = 195). The average sample size was 173, ranging from 78 to 491 participants. All 6 studies included in this review used a pretest/posttest design. The geographic regions included Australia (n = 2), Canada (n = 1), China (n = 1), Taiwan (n = 1), and the United States (n = 1).[13–18] Five of the 6 studies received a GRADE of "moderate" indicating lower risk of bias, inconsistencies, and imprecision.[13,14,16–18] One study received a "low" GRADE due to a smaller sample size, lack of randomization, and risk for publication bias.[15] Studies included in this review did not receive "high" GRADE ratings due to comparatively smaller sample sizes and lack of representation from diverse gender and ethnic groups. The researchers discovered 3 recurring themes related to using simulation-based learning to illustrate pain: compassionate communication, interprofessional collaboration, and advocacy for vulnerable populations.

Compassionate Communication

Compassionate care and communication are recognized as crucial concepts for nursing practice by the American Association of College of Nursing, both encompassing respectful and empathetic interactions with patients who are further emphasized in Domain 2: Person-Centered Care and Domain 9: Professionalism.[10] Compassionate care is a union of empathy and a nurse's desire to alleviate patient suffering, address individualized care needs, and use of therapeutic communication with patients.[19] Clear and concise communication forms the foundation that builds bridges and forges relationships.[20] Person-centered communication and interactions are imperative to compassionate care.[20]

This review of the literature revealed that compassionate communication was a common outcome for using simulation to illustrate pain. All studies (n = 6) included in this review directly or indirectly measured compassionate communication through being attuned to nonverbal cues, having a considerate attitude, using empathetic language,

Table 1
Table of evidence

Author	Location	Model	Methodology	Intervention	Participants	Population	Variables	Instruments	Results	GRADE
Chu et al,[13] 2019	Taiwan	Addie Model	Quasi-experimental pretest/posttest	Screen based	New nurses	Unknown	Satisfaction knowledge ability	New Nurse Pain Care Satisfaction Pain Care Knowledge Scale Pain Care Ability Appraisal	The experimental group had higher satisfaction scores and demonstrated greater knowledge of pain assessment. New comers in the experimental group also had better communication to perform a pain assessment.	Moderate
Kang et al,[14] 2022	China	N/A	Quasi experimental	Standardized patients	New nurses	65 year old man 65 year old woman 80 year old man	Knowledge skill Critical thinking satisfaction	Knowledge Questionnaire Clinical Evaluation California Critical Thinking Disposition Inventory Learning Satisfaction Scale	The simulation group was significantly greater in knowledge of pain management, and knowledge of special scenario communication, and the skill score of turnovers than the control group. The critical-thinking score was also greater in the simulation group. The simulation group had a higher satisfaction in learning.	Moderate

(continued on next page)

Table 1
(continued)

Author	Location	Model	Methodology	Intervention	Participants	Population	Variables	Instruments	Results	GRADE
Kelly et al,[15] 2022	Australia	Tanner's Clinical Judgment Model	Exploratory mixed methods pretest/posttest	Screen based	Nursing students	Chinese male patient who spoke little English with daughter for interpretation	Compassion noticing interpreting	Compassion Scale Lasater Clinical Judgment Rubric	The majority of participants were able to identify that the patient was in greater pain than self-reported. Some participants were unable to notice and interpret the impact of culture during pain assessment. Participants were more aware of the subjectivity of pain and that the strategies learned from this activity would improve future clinical practice.	Low
Kelly et al,[16] 2024	Australia	Strobe	Descriptive pretest/posttest	Screen based	Nursing students	Differences in gender, age, and chronic vs acute pain	Compassion feasibility relevance	Compassion Scale Investigator-Developed Surveys	The simulations were easy to understand, relevant to practice, and beneficial in prompting reflection on patient's responses to pain and nurses' critical thinking. Compassion scores increased significantly following the	Moderate

Simko et al,[17] 2021	United States	N/A	Quasi-experimental pretest/posttest	Wearable devices	IPE students	Individual with chronic pain	Empathy	Jefferson Scale of Empathy-Health Professions Scale Kiersma-Chen Empathy Scale	Scores from the empathy scales indicate the use of the kit significantly increased empathy in pharmacy, nursing, and health science students.	Moderate
Watt-Watson et al,[18] 2019	Canada	N/A	Prospective pretest/posttest	Screen based	IPE students	Diverse gender and ethnic patients with progressive acute to chronic pain	Design usability knowledge beliefs assessment	Design and Usability Survey Pain Knowledge and Beliefs Pain Assessment Skills Tool (PAST)	Overall usability scores were strong, pain knowledge scores increased 20%. The PAST was sensitive to differences in student level of experience but was an effective tool for delivering formative feedback.	Moderate

exuding kindness, and being cognizant of the patient's beliefs.[13–18] Chu and colleagues[13] indirectly assessed the compassionate communication of new nursing graduates following a computer-based pain simulation and found that scores were significantly higher for the experimental group than the control group. These results were assessed using the Pain Care Ability Appraisal.[13] Kang and colleagues[14] also found similar results in compassionate communication using standardized patients as the simulation modality. The studies included in this review that directly assessed compassion utilized the Compassion Scale and found that simulation-based learning was an effective educational strategy for improving self-perceptions of compassion.[15,16,21]

Interprofessional Collaboration

Interprofessional collaboration is an intentional partnership across professions that includes the nurse, patient, family, and multiple other health care disciplines (eg, medicine, occupational therapy, physical therapy, pharmacy). These partnerships enhance health care experiences and strengthen patient outcomes.[10] Interprofessional collaboration aligns with Domain 6: Interprofessional Partnerships of the Core Competencies for Professional Nursing Education.[10] Additionally, the IASP identifies interprofessional collaboration as an essential part of the curriculum for teaching pain in nursing.[11] Nurses are expected to exhibit effective collaboration as interprofessional team members to develop and define realistic and mutual goals for pain management.[11] This review revealed 2 studies that focused on interprofessional collaboration for training students in pain management.[17,18]

Simko and colleagues[17] conducted a pretest/posttest study to evaluate the changes in empathy among pharmacy, nursing, and health sciences students following a Chronic Pain Simulation Empathy Training Kit. The simulation training provided an immersive experiential learning experience in which wearable devices were applied before completing activities of daily living. This simulation-based learning opportunity was offered in an elective interprofessional course.[17] Empathy was measured using the Jefferson Scale of Empathy-Health Professions Scale (JSE-HPS) and the Kiersma-Chen Empathy Scale (KCES). Composite JSE-HPS and KCES empathy scores increased by 5.83 and 5.91 points, respectively ($P<.00001$).[17]

Watt-Watson and colleagues[18] developed a similar interprofessional elective course incorporating screen-based simulation using the IASP interprofessional curriculum standards. Participants in this study were students in pharmacy, nursing, dentistry, medicine, occupational therapy, physical therapy, pharmacy, and social work. The Pain Knowledge and Beliefs tool measured beliefs related to pain mechanisms, assessment, and management. Participants demonstrated a 20.6% increase in pain knowledge and beliefs ($P<.00001$).[18] While not specifically developed to assess interprofessional collaboration, Kang and colleagues[14] found that simulation-based learning with standardized patients increased students' satisfaction and attitudes toward working in an interprofessional health care team.

Advocacy for Vulnerable Populations

Previous research has found that the most significant impact of pain occurs among the geriatric population, female individuals, adults living in poverty, and those living in rural areas.[1] Nurses are instrumental in providing care to ensure equitable health outcomes for all patient populations with attention and advocacy for the most vulnerable populations.[10] The IASP stresses the importance of providing pain education related to social factors such as cultural differences, family dynamics, language barriers, gender, age, and ethnicity.[11] Additionally, nurses must be trained on the barriers to achieving pain management with those who are cognitively impaired, critically ill, and nonverbal.[11]

The majority (n = 5) of studies included in this review utilized simulation-based learning scenarios that portrayed vulnerable populations.[14–18] Patients varied by age, gender, and socioeconomic status, with differences in diagnosis, language barriers, and presence of support. Kelly and colleagues[15] utilized a screen-based simulation to portray a Chinese male patient who spoke little English but used his daughter for interpretation. While some students did not notice and interpret the impact of culture during the pain assessment, others recognized that cultural aspects led to difficult communication and masking of pain.[15] Kang and colleagues[14] utilized standardized patients to illustrate palliative care in the Chinese culture, historically known for opposition to the conversation and care associated with death. This cultural stigma related to death leads to poorly educated health care professionals caring for patients receiving palliative care. Using simulation to illustrate pain in this vulnerable population significantly increased knowledge of pain management, communication, critical thinking, and skill with greater satisfaction in learning.[14]

DISCUSSION

The results show that using simulation-based learning to illustrate pain can increase learner satisfaction, knowledge, clinical judgment, compassion, and empathy in nursing and interprofessional teams. The studies included in this review utilized different modalities; however, most studies (n = 4) provided the patient scenario through a screen-based multimedia platform. The primary use of screen-based simulations raises the question if modality influences learner outcomes. We question whether differences would occur between the use of high-fidelity mannequins, screen-based simulations, and standardized patient scenarios. While the IASP provides curricular guidelines for pain education,[11] only one study utilized the curriculum resources provided by the IASP.[18] This raises the question of the number of educational and health care institutions that utilize the IASP curricular guidelines for training. We see the benefit of utilizing these resources to strengthen current curricular structures and workforce training. Providing a standardized training curriculum for health care professionals further promotes interprofessional collaboration in turn improving patient-centered care.

SUMMARY

This article aims to determine the current evidence related to using simulation-based learning for training and teaching the assessment and management of pain in the nursing discipline. A review of the literature discovered that simulation-based learning can be an effective educational strategy to encourage compassionate communication, interprofessional collaboration, and advocacy for vulnerable populations. We encourage health care educators and practicing clinicians to use this knowledge to incorporate education related to pain into future and existing curriculum structures with simulation-based learning as the method of instruction. Furthermore, we encourage interprofessional simulation-based learning experiences to enhance opportunities for collaborative partnerships and to improve quality of patient care.

CLINICS CARE POINTS

- The IASP provides curriculum outlines to introduce the knowledge and skills needed to assess and manage pain.

- Simulation is an effective educational strategy to encourage compassionate communication, interprofessional collaboration, and advocacy for vulnerable populations.
- Using simulation to illustrate pain can increase learner satisfaction, knowledge, clinical judgment, compassion, and empathy in nursing and interprofessional teams.

DISCLOSURE

There are no financial conflicts of interest to disclose.

REFERENCES

1. Rikard SM, Strahan AE, Schmit KM, et al. Chronic pain among adults - United States, 2019-2021. MMWR Morbidity Mortality Weekly Report 2023;72(15).
2. Nahin RL, Feinberg T, Kapos FP, et al. Estimated rates of incident and persistent chronic pain among US adults, 2019-2020. JAMA Netw Open 2023;6(5):e2313563.
3. Pilcher J, Goodall H, Jensen C, et al. Special focus on simulation: educational strategies in the NICU: simulation-based learning: it's not just for NRP. Neonatal Netw 2012;31(5):281–7.
4. Immonen K, Oikarainen A, Tomietto M, et al. Assessment of nursing students' competence in clinical practice: a systematic review of reviews. Int J Nurs Stud 2019;100:103414.
5. Keddington AS, Moore J. Simulation as a method of competency assessment among health care providers: a systematic review. Nurs Educ Perspect 2019; 40(2):91–4.
6. Kiernan LC. Evaluating competence and confidence using simualtion technology. Nursing 2018;48(10):45–52.
7. Kim S, Lee H, Connerton TP. How psychological safety affects team performance: mediating role of efficacy and learning behavior. Front Psychol 2020;11:1581.
8. Madireddy S, Rufa EP. Maintaining confidentiality and psychological safety in medical simulation, . StatPearls. StatPearls Publishing; 2023. Available at: https://www.ncbi.nlm.nih.gov/books/NBK559259/. [Accessed 21 February 2024].
9. INACSL Standards Committee. Onward and upward: introducing the healthcare simulation standards of best practice™. Clinical Simulation in Nursing 2021; 58:1–4.
10. American Association of Colleges of Nursing (AACN). The essentials: Core competencies for professional nursing edcuation. 2021. Available at: https://www.aacnnursing.org/Portals/42/AcademicNursing/pdf/Essentials-2021.pdf. [Accessed 16 January 2024].
11. International association for the study of pain (IASP). Curriculum outline on pain for nursing. 2018. Available at: https://www.iasp-pain.org/education/curricula/iasp-curriculum-outline-on-pain-for-nursing/. [Accessed 16 January 2024].
12. Guyatt GH, Oxman AD, Vist GE, et al. GRADE: an emerging consensus on rating quality of evidence and strength of recommendations. BMJ 2008;336(7650): 924–6.
13. Chu TL, Wang J, Lin HL, et al. Multimedia-assisted instruction on pain assessment learning of new nurses: a quasi-experimental study. BMC Med Educ 2019;19(1):68.
14. Kang D, Zhang L, Jin S, et al. Effectiveness of palliative care simulation in newly hired oncology nurses' training. Asia Pac J Oncol Nurs 2022;9(3):167–73.

15. Kelly MA, Slatyer S, Myers H, et al. Using audio-visual simulation to elicit nursing students' noticing and interpreting skills to assess pain in culturally diverse patients. Clinical Simulation in Nursing 2022;71:31–40.

16. Kelly MA, Slatyer S, Tutticci N, et al. Challenging the nuances of pain assessment with co-designed audio-visual simulations in nursing education: a descriptive study. Clinical Simulation in Nursing 2024;87:101510.

17. Simko LC, Rhodes DC, Gumireddy A, et al. Effects of a chronic pain simulation empathy training kit on the empathy of interprofessional healthcare students for chronic pain patients. Clinical Simulation in Nursing 2021;56:66–75.

18. Watt-Watson J, McGillion M, Lax L, et al. Evaluating an innovative elearning pain education interprofessional resource: a pre-post study. Pain Med 2019;20(1): 37–49.

19. Su JJ, Masika GM, Paguio JT, et al. Defining compassionate nursing care. Nurs Ethics 2020;27(2):480–93.

20. Chaloner RSF. Providing compassionate care for every kind of person. J Healthc Manag 2019;64(4):205–8.

21. Pommier E, Neff KD, Tóth-Király I. The development and validation of the compassion scale. Assessment 2020;27(1):21–39.

Management of Neonatal Pain Associated with Circumcision

Teresa Ellett, DNP, MSN, BSN, RN, CNE[a],*,
Lisa Wallace, DNP, MSN, RN, RNC-OB, NE-BC[b]

KEYWORDS

- Circumcision • Circumcision care • Pain management • Newborns
- Pain assessment • Analgesia

KEY POINTS

- Newborns experience pain during and post circumcision.
- Providing local or topical analgesia measures may decrease the pain associated with circumcision.
- Adequate training is needed to improve the scoring of neonatal pain using available pain scales.
- The role of the nurse includes teaching the family how to care for and comfort the newborn after a circumcision.

BACKGROUND

Neonatal circumcision is a painful procedure often performed on male newborns within the first few days of life. There has been controversy over the years about newborn pain associated with circumcision; however, providing analgesia during the procedure has become customary practice.[1] Addressing newborn pain during painful procedures is essential to avoid harmful long-term effects.[2] The reader is referred to **Box 1** outlining the acute and potential long-term consequences associated with untreated pain in infants.[2] Providing analgesia to alleviate pain with procedures needs to be a standard part of neonatal care.[3]

The decision of whether to have a male circumcised may be influenced by a variety of factors such as religious or cultural beliefs, and medical reasons.[4] The American Academy of Pediatrics found that circumcision may have the following advantages: a lower risk of penile cancer, lower risk of human immunodeficiency virus, and lower

[a] Morehead State University, 316 West Second Street, 201K Center for Health, Education, and Research, Morehead, KY 40351, USA; [b] Morehead State University, 316 West Second Street, 201D Center for Health, Education, and Research, Morehead, KY 40351, USA
* Corresponding author.
E-mail address: t.ellett@moreheadstate.edu

Crit Care Nurs Clin N Am 36 (2024) 517–530
https://doi.org/10.1016/j.cnc.2024.04.010
ccnursing.theclinics.com

> **Box 1**
> **Consequences of untreated pain in infants**
>
> Acute Consequences
>   Periventricular-intraventricular hemorrhage
>   Increased chemical and hormone release
>   Breakdown of fat and carbohydrate stores
>   Prolonged hyperglycemia
>   Higher morbidity for neonatal intensive care unit patients
>   Memory of painful events
>   Hypersensitivity to pain
>   Prolonged response to pain
>   Inappropriate innervation of the spinal cord
>   Inappropriate response to nonnoxious stimuli
>   Lower pain threshold
>
> Potential Long-Term Consequences
>   Higher somatic complaints of unknown origin
>   Greater physiologic and behavioral responses to pain
>   Increased prevalence of neurologic deficits
>   Psychosocial problems
>   Neurobehavioral disorders
>   Cognitive deficits
>   Learning disorders
>   Poor motor performance
>   Behavioral problems
>   Attention deficits
>   Poor adaptive behavior
>   Inability to cope with novel situations
>   Problems with impulsivity and social control
>   Learning deficits
>   Emotional temperament changes in infancy or childhood
>   Accentuated hormonal stress response in adult life
>
> *Data from* Hockenberry MJ. Pain assessment and management in children. In: Perry SE, Lowder-milk DL, Cashion K, Alden KR, Olshansky EF, and Hockenberry MJ. Maternal child nursing care, 7th edition. St Louis: Elsevier; 2023. p. 781.

sexually transmitted infections for males.[5] Some parents may choose not to circumcise their infant; however, 10% to 15% of uncircumcised newborns will require a circumcision later in life due to penile complications.[6] The purpose of this manuscript is to share information on circumcision care, procedural pain management, and education provided to the family.

Circumcision

The national rate of circumcisions performed on newborns in the hospital setting decreased from approximately 65% to 58% during 1979 to 2010.[7] Circumcision is not considered a routine procedure and is ultimately decided upon by the parents unless contraindicated.[5] One study found that men who are circumcised often choose to circumcise their healthy male newborns.[8] Circumcision should not be performed on some male newborns for reasons that are contraindicated including bleeding disorders, congenital anomalies, and insufficient size of the penis.[9]

Parents may choose to have their newborns circumcised before discharge from the hospital after delivery. Providers are required to discuss the risks and benefits associated with circumcision with parents prior to obtaining informed consent. When discussing consent with the provider, parents need to ask questions about pain control measures that will be used during the procedure.

TYPES OF CIRCUMCISION INSTRUMENTS

The type of device used for performing the newborn circumcision may impact the level of pain experienced by the newborn during the procedure. There are a variety of devices used for newborn circumcision including the Gomco (**Fig. 1**A),[10] Mogen (**Fig. 1**B),[10] and Plastibell based upon practitioner preference.[4,11] The Mogen is the quickest method (12 minutes) when used by trained experts compared to the Plastibell (**Fig. 2**)[10] which took the longest (20 minutes).[11] Research showed that using a Mogen device while performing a circumcision led to lower pain scores in newborns than using other devices.[4] Ultimately, the type of device used is at the discretion of the provider performing the procedure.

PATHOPHYSIOLOGY OF PAIN

Gestational age, illness severity, and the repetitiveness of painful procedures may affect a newborn's response to pain.[12] The International Association for the Study of Pain as cited in Raja and colleagues defines pain as "An unpleasant sensory and emotional experience that is associated with actual or potential tissue damage or described in terms of such damage" (p. 1976).[13] The newborn's brain weight almost triples during the first year of life, as the nervous system continues to mature and achieve all cortical and brain stem cells.[14] Neurologic development occurs in a cephalocaudal and proximal-distal pattern and pain is highly individualized (p. 592).[14] According to the American College of Obstetricians and Gynecologists, a fetus can feel pain after 24 weeks intrauterine development.[15] Further Tobias found that preterm infants experience pain at a greater level due to the lack of inhibitory responses that result from central nervous system development as infants age (qtd. in Ricci, Kyle & Carmen 1248).[14]

Pain involves special nerve endings (nociceptors) which are activated by noxious stimuli such as mechanical, chemical, and thermal which cause various transduction reactions. Mechanical may cause intense pressure in an area or muscle stretching, whereas chemical causes release of mediators, including histamine, prostaglandins, leukotrienes, or bradykinin, related to tissue trauma, ischemia, or inflammation.[14]

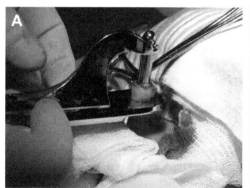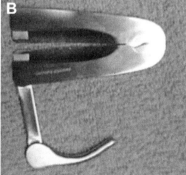

Fig. 1. (*A* and *B*) Circumcision. (*A*) Gomco. (*B*) The Mogen clamp. (*From* Alden KR. Nursing Care of the Newborn and Family. In: Perry SE, Lowdermilk DL, Cashion K, Alden KR, Olshansky EF, and Hockenberry MJ. Maternal Child Nursing Care, 7th edition. St Louis: Elsevier; 2023. p. 566. https://evolve.elsevier.com/cs/product/9780323776714?role=student. (Image Courtesy: [*A*] Cheryl Briggs, RNC, Annapolis, MD. [*B*] Patricia A. Scott, Nashville, TN).)

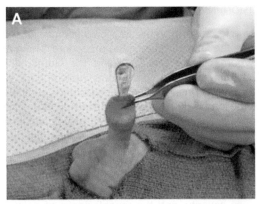

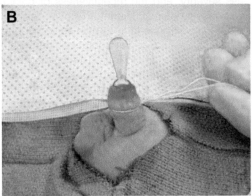

Fig. 2. Plastibell. (*A*) Plastibell is positioned over the glans. (*B*) A string is secured around the penis in the slot of the bell. The extra foreskin is cut off and handle removed from the bell. (*Data from* Alden KR. Nursing Care of the Newborn and Family. In: Perry SE, Lowdermilk DL, Cashion K, Alden KR, Olshansky EF, and Hockenberry MJ. Maternal Child Nursing Care, 7th edition. St Louis: Elsevier; 2023. p. 566. https://evolve.elsevier.com/cs/product/9780323776714?role=student. *From* Holocomb, G.W. Murphy, J.P. Ostile, D. J. [2014] Ashcraft's pediatric surgery [6th ed.] Philadelphia: Elsevier)

Thermal is related to very hot or cold stimuli.[14] Next, these transduction reactions are converted to electrical impulses that travel along the peripheral nerves to the central nervous system (spinal cord and brain) transmitted through neurotransmitters to the dorsal horn of the spinal cord that split up toward the thalamus.[14] The thalamus sends messages to the somatosensory part of the brain which interprets the physical sensation of pain.[14] The A-delta fibers respond to sharp, stabbing localized pain leading to a rapid reflex to withdraw from the stimulus and C fibers that lead to the perception of a diffuse, dull, burning, or aching pain.[14] The pain threshold is the point of lowest intensity of a painful stimulus. The thalamus also sends a message to the Limbic system that activates emotions and autonomic nervous system to react, such as changes in vital signs or the *fight or flight reaction*.[14] Pain may be modified centrally at the dorsal horn or peripherally by neuromodulators, which may include serotonin, endorphins, enkephalins, and dynorphins which may block or change perception of pain.[14]

Pain may have an acute or chronic onset and the duration may be continuous or intermittent.[14] Pain is influenced by various environmental, emotional, or physiologic factors.[14] Nociceptive pain affects primarily tissues which may also be described as somatic pain, whereas neuropathic pain is related to the peripheral or central nervous system. Visceral pain is related to organ pain. Descriptive words for pain may include sharp, burning, dull, aching, squeezing, radiating, spasm-like, cramping, or stabbing.[14] Pain is also influenced by gender, age, experiences, cognitive level, family, culture, temperament, and situational factors.[14]

PAIN ASSESSMENT

Pain assessment is an essential role of the nurse caring for newborns scheduled to have painful procedures. It is more difficult to assess the pain level of newborns due to their inability to provide verbal feedback.[16] Nurses must rely on their ability to assess physiologic and behavioral changes associated with newborn pain. The reader is referred to **Box 2** for physiologic and behavioral manifestations of acute pain in the neonate.[10] Physiologic responses to pain include alterations in vital signs, oxygenation, skin, laboratory evidence of metabolic or endocrine changes, and other observations.[10] Behavioral responses to pain include variations in vocalizations, facial expression, body movements, and posture and changes in state.[10] Therefore, pain may be measured by monitoring vital signs, pulse oximetry, sweating of palms, vagal tone, crying, motor activity, and facial expressions of pain.[17] Facial signs of discomfort in a newborn are shown in **Fig. 3**.[10]

Pain assessment scales are beneficial for assessing the newborn's pain level.[18] However, a systematic review conducted by Garcia-Rodriguez et al. found that nurses may not fully understand how to interpret pain scales used in assessing neonatal pain associated with painful procedures.[19] It would be beneficial for nurses to receive additional training improving their use of these scales.[19] There are many different pain assessment scales that may be utilized to effectively assess the pain level of newborns. Providers and nurses may use the pain scales listed in **Table 1** to assess and evaluate newborn pain with circumcision.[20–25]

In a cross-sectional study, neonatal intensive care unit nurses reported that they witnessed physiologic indicators and behavioral changes more often than certain facial expressions associated with pain.[18] These nurses denied using pain assessment scales on a routine basis. Recommendations were providing nurses with more education related to assessing and managing the pain of critically ill neonates and implementing guidelines for practice.[18]

PHARMACOLOGIC PAIN MANAGEMENT

Pain management during circumcision is inconsistent from one practitioner to another.[26] Even though research suggests that circumcision causes pain for the newborn during the procedure, providers do not always administer adequate analgesia.[12] On the other hand, a trained licensed health care provider may order additional pre-operative medications to decrease pain experienced during the procedure. There are several common methods used to provide pain control during circumcision.[4] Pharmacologic interventions may include acetaminophen, fentanyl, lidocaine, or eutectic mixture of local anesthetics (EMLA) cream.[4] Other pharmacologic measures include oral sucrose (24% solution), systemic drugs like nonsteroidal anti-inflammatory drugs, opioids, or general anesthetics.[27]

Dorsal penile nerve block (DPNB) and lidocaine-prilocaine cream (LPC) are commonly used analgesics prior to circumcision.[28] EMLA with 2.5% lidocaine and 2.5% prilocaine cream may be applied to the skin around the penis, covered with a transparent dressing for at least 1 to 1 1/2 hours before the procedure takes place

Box 2
Manifestations of acute pain in the newborn

- Physiologic Responses
  - Vital signs
  - Increased heart rate
  - Increased blood pressure
  - Rapid, shallow respirations

- Oxygenation
  - Decreased transcutaneous oxygen saturation
  - Decreased arterial oxygen saturation

- Skin
  - Pallor or flushing
  - Diaphoresis
  - Palmar sweating

- Laboratory evidence of metabolic or endocrine changes
  - Hyperglycemia
  - Lowered pH
  - Elevated corticosteroids

- Other observations
  - Increased muscle tone
  - Dilated pupils
  - Decreased vagal nerve tone
  - Increased intracranial pressure

- Behavioral Responses

- Vocalizations
  - Crying
  - Whimpering
  - Groaning

- Facial expression
  - Grimace
  - Brow furrowed
  - Chin quivering
  - Eyes tightly closed
  - Mouth open and squarish

- Body movements and posture
  - Limb withdrawal
  - Thrashing
  - Rigidity
  - Flaccidity
  - Fist clenching

- Changes in state
  - Changes in sleep-wake cycles
  - Changes in feeding behavior
  - Changes in activity level
  - Fussiness, irritability
  - Listlessness

Data from Alden KR. Nursing Care of the Newborn and Family. In: Perry SE, Lowdermilk DL, Cashion K, Alden KR, Olshansky EF, and Hockenberry MJ. Maternal Child Nursing Care, 7th edition. St Louis: Elsevier; 2023. p. 568.

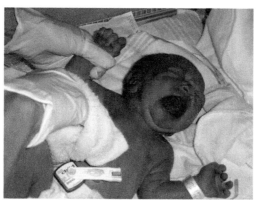

Fig. 3. Signs of pain in the newborn. (*Data from* Alden KR. Nursing Care of the Newborn and Family. In: Perry SE, Lowdermilk DL, Cashion K, Alden KR, Olshansky EF, and Hockenberry MJ. Maternal Child Nursing Care, 7th edition. St Louis: Elsevier; 2023. p. 567. https://evolve.elsevier.com/cs/product/9780323776714?role=student. *Courtesy* Kathryn Alden, Stanley, NC)

without combining with another method.[1] Application of LPC prior to the DPNB was found to reduce the pain associated with administering the DPNB and provided more pain control during the Plastibell circumcision procedure than using a DPNB exclusively.[28] Administering a DPNB requires the newborn to be secured on a restraint board with arms and legs restrained (**Fig. 4**).[10] One disadvantage is that using LPC does require an extended waiting period to allow for the medication to take effect. One study cited that use of the DPNB was 100% effective in reducing pain in 70% of circumcisions.[11] A meta-analysis of reducing neonatal pain during procedures recommends a dual approach with oral sucrose and non-nutritive suckling, such as with a pacifier.[29]

A prospective randomized clinical trial found that when both EMLA and sucrose were used during circumcision, the pain scores of newborns were significantly lower than that of using only 1 of them.[12] One study concluded that the DPNB was more effective in providing pain relief during circumcision than using the EMLA cream alone.[30] A pilot study found that newborns had significantly lower pain scores based upon the Face, Legs, Activity, Cry and Consolability pain scale when analgesia combined with oral sucrose was used for newborn circumcision.[26]

Another research study cited that bupivacaine 0.5% was found more effective than 1% lidocaine for DPNB.[31] In 2023, a research study was performed assessing neonatal circumcision pain administering oral ketamine 10 mg/kg (weight) suggesting additional future research for validation.[32] Research supports use of analgesics with other combined interventions resulting in more long-term benefits for the pediatric patient.[33] One study supports combining local anesthesia and analgesia with lidocaine-prilocaine cream and use of the Mogen clamp to reduce circumcision pain.[34]

NON-PHARMACOLOGICAL MANAGEMENT

Many nonpharmacological and pharmacologic pain control interventions have been adopted over time.[27] Nonpharmacological management consists of the following: "breastfeeding or expressed breast milk, skin to skin contact or kangaroo mother care , swaddling, and non-nutritive sucking (NNS), among others" (p.1).[27] **Fig. 5** shows

Table 1
Summary of pain assessment scales for infants

	PIPP-Revised (Stevens, Gibbins Yamada, et al,[21] 2014)	Neonatal Infant Pain Scale (Lawrence, Alcock, McGrath, et al,[22] 1993)	Neonatal Pain Agitation and Sedation Scale (N-Pass) (Hummel, Puchalski, Creech, et al,[23] 2008)	COMFORT-Neo (van Dijk, Roofthooft, Anand, et al,[24] 2009)	CRIES (Krechel & Bildner, 1996)
Age Range	25–40 wk	26–40 wk	23–40 wk	24–42 wk	32–40 wk
Type of Pain	Procedural and postoperative		Procedural and prolonged	Prolonged pain	Postoperative pain
Variables Assessed	Scored at (0–3) each Heart rate Oxygen saturation Brow bulge Eye squeeze Nasolabial furrow Behavioral state	Breathing (0–1) Face (0–1) Arms (0–1) Legs (0–1) Cry (0–2) Arousal (0–1)	Scored at (0–2) each Vital signs Crying/irritability Facial expressions Behavioral state Extremities/tone	Scored at (1–5) each Alertness Calmness/agitation Respiratory response or crying Body movement Muscle tone Facial tension	Scored at (0–2) each Crying Oxygen requirement Changes to vital signs Facial expressions Sleeplessness
Score Range	0–21	0–7	Pain (1–10)	6–30	0–10
Adjusted for Gestational Age	Yes Scored at (0–3)	No	Yes	No	No

Abbreviations: CRIES, crying, requiring increased oxygen, increased vital signs, expression, and sleeplessness; NIPS, neonatal infant pain scal; PIPP- revised, premature infant pain scale.
Data from Hellsten MB. Pain Assessment in Children. In: Hockenberry, MJ., Duffy EA, & Gibbs KD, Wong's Nursing Care of Infants and children, 12th edition. St. Louis: Elsevier; 2024. p. 139.

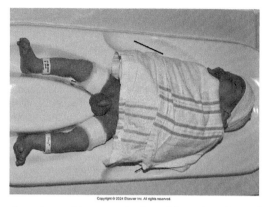

Fig. 4. Infant secured on circumcision restraint board for safety. (*Data from* Wallace L. Care of the Newborn. In: Murray S, McKinney E, Holub KS, Jones R, and Scheffer KL. Foundations of Maternal-Newborn and Women's Health Nursing, 8th edition. St Louis: Elsevier; 2023. p. 617.)

an infant being swaddled and using non-nutritive sucking to provide comfort following a circumcision.[10] NNS was believed to be associated with antinociceptive mechanisms and sucrose appears to enhance the effect of NNS, leading to an increase of endogenous endorphins.[35] Audio stimulation with music may also be beneficial in

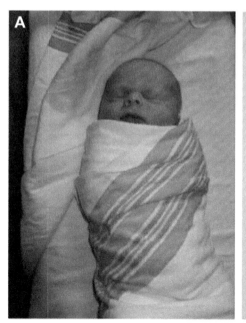
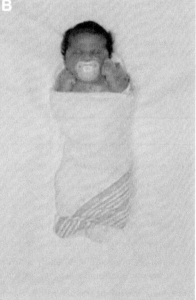

Fig. 5. (*A* and *B*) Swaddling. (*A*) Newborn swaddled for comfort. (*B*) An infant being swaddled and using nonnutritive sucking to provide comfort following a circumcision. (*Data from* Alden KR. Nursing Care of the Newborn and Family. In: Perry SE, Lowdermilk DL, Cashion K, Alden KR, Olshansky EF, and Hockenberry MJ. Maternal Child Nursing Care, 7th edition. St Louis: Elsevier; 2023. p. 568. https://evolve.elsevier.com/cs/product/9780323776714?role=student. [*A*] *Courtesy* of Jennifer and Travis Alderman, Durham, NC. [*B*] *Courtesy* Cheryl Briggs, RNC, Annapolis, MD.)

Box 3
Sample circumcision order set

Sample Circumcision Order Set
1. Obtain Informed Consent
2. Pre-procedure (optional as ordered per licensed health care provider) (at least 30 minutes)
   Acetaminophen oral suspension 30 minutes before procedure
   Weight: _____g 10 mg/kg/dose – OR– ☐ 15 mg/kg/dose.
3. Apply topical EMLA/lidocaine cream to circumcision site 30 to 60 minutes before the procedure and cover loosely with clear, bioocclusive dressing to avoid diaper absorption (see manufacturer's instructions).
4. Cover circumcision board with warmed blanket and place infant gently securing straps per manufacturer's instructions and maintaining newborn warmth. Staff member or family/guardian support will remain at bedside once placed on board until post-procedure placement back into crib, bassinette, or parent/guardian arms.
5. Intra-operative Dorsal Penile Nerve block administered per licensed health care provider:
   ☐ 0.5% bupivacaine—OR— ☐ 1% lidocaine
6. Sucrose solution: Offer a sucrose solution to the infant during the procedure for its analgesic effect. Dose: Administer 24% sucrose solution orally per licensed health care provider orders before the procedure.
7. Provide non-nutritive suckling via a pacifier or gloved finger during the procedure.
8. Provide soothing touch or quiet, soothing sound or music during the procedure.
9. Post-procedure:
   • ☐ Acetaminophen oral suspension: Provide for pain if not done pre-procedure.
     Dose: Administer ____mg/kg/dose (weight) oral suspension every 4 to 6 hours as needed for pain.
   • Monitor site every 15 minutes for the first hour for bleeding, discharge, swelling, or voiding; may need to extend monitoring time if actively bleeding.
   • Provide comfort measures such as cuddling, breastfeeding (if applicable), gentle rocking, skin-to-skin/kangaroo care to soothe the infant.
   • Avoid tight clothing or diapers that may cause friction or irritation to the circumcision site.
   • Observe for infant voiding within 6 to 8 hours with adequate oral intake.
10. Notify the provider for the following:
    • Increased bleeding
    • Inability to void
    • Signs of infection (temperature >100.5° Fahrenheit, redness, swelling, or malodorous drainage)

Box 4
Basic care and comfort for circumcision

1. Provide a quiet environment.
2. This is a sterile procedure. Have the correct size for surgical gloves used by the provider.
3. Apply a topical anesthetic prior to the procedure as ordered by the provider.
4. Apply a topical analgesic as ordered by the provider.
5. Keep area dry and then apply petroleum jelly liberally to prevent skin irritation (Do not apply petroleum jelly if a Plastibell is used).
6. Expect the infant to void within 6 to 8 hours of the procedure.
7. Expect the infant to cry after the first void following the procedure.
8. Clean the area with water daily, and whenever the area becomes soiled with a bowel movement.
9. Expect the scab that forms post-procedure to fall off 2-week post procedure.
10. Provide care information to parents and answer posed questions.

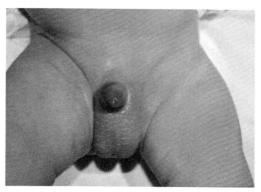

Fig. 6. Circumcised newborn. (*Data from* McKinney ES, Murray SS, Mau K, James SR, Nelson KA, Ashwill JW, & Carroll J. Maternal-child nursing, 6th edition. St. Louis: Elsevier; 2022. p. 479. *Courtesy* Cheryl Briggs, RNC, Annapolis, MD.)

reducing pain.[4] One study reported that having the parent or caregiver present supported providing the pediatric patient a calmer environment leading to less stress/anxiety and pain.[33] If a parent or caregiver is not able to be present, a Child Life Specialist may be available who is trained in the primary role of reducing pain and stress.[33]

BASIC CARE AND COMFORT PRE-CIRCUMCISION AND POST-CIRCUMCISION

The provider and nursing staff will employ basic care and comfort measures. A study by Qahtani suggested that hospitals establish and put into effect circumcision protocols with a goal of improving the pain management of newborns.[12] **Box 3** shows a sample order set that may be used as a guide in protocol or policy development. Providing parents with education on how to be actively involved in comforting their baby after painful procedures is a significant role of the nurse.[18] The reader is referred to **Box 4** to learn steps in the circumcision procedure and care interventions during and post procedure.

SUMMARY

Circumcision is an elective, surgical procedure commonly performed on newborns. **Fig. 6** shows a newborn who has recently been circumcised.[36] Research supports that repetitive exposure to painful procedures from birth through early childhood may negatively impact cognitive, motor, and neurologic development.[37] Therefore, it is imperative that providers use analgesia and pain control interventions to reduce the pain and stress caused by circumcision. At this point in time, a standardized approach to pain management has not been established. Additional research is needed to determine the best analgesia for use during circumcision. Furthermore, it would be beneficial for facilities to adopt a policy or procedure specific to pain control of newborns during circumcision.

CLINICS CARE POINTS

- Several pain scales are available to assess newborn pain associated with circumcision.
- Protocols/policies are beneficial to guide providers and nurses with managing newborn pain in the health care setting.

- Providers and nurses need to be familiar with pharmacologic and nonpharmacological measures to address newborn pain with circumcision.
- A significant role of the nurse is to educate parents on the ways to comfort their newborn after a circumcision.

DISCLOSURE

All authors report no commercial or financial conflicts of interest. There was no funding from any source for this publication.

REFERENCES

1. Rossi S, Buonocore G, Bellieni CV. Management of pain in newborn circumcision: a systematic review. Eur J Pediatr 2021;180:13–20.
2. Hockenberry MJ. Pain assessment and management in children. In: Perry SE, Lowdermilk DL, Cashion K, et al, editors. Maternal child nursing care. 7th edition. St Louis: Elsevier; 2023. p. 781.
3. Ponder BL. Effects of pain in the human neonate. Am J END Technol 2002;42: 210–23.
4. Bellieni CV, Alagna MG, Buonocore G. Analgesia for infants' circumcision. Ital J Pediatr 2013;39:38. Available at: http://jponline.net.content/39/1/38.
5. Blank S, Brady M, Buerk E, et al. Circumcision policy statement. Pediatrics 2012; 130(3):585–6.
6. International Childbirth Education Association. ICEA position statement and review: neonatal circumcision. Int J Civ Eng 2002;17:3.
7. Centers for Disease Control and Prevention. Trends in circumcision for male newborns in U.S. hospitals:1979-2010. 2015. Available at: https://www.cdc.gov/nchs/data/hestat/circumcision_2013/circumcision_2013.htm.
8. Guevara CG, Achua JK, Blachman-Braun R, et al. Neonatal circumcision: what are the factors affecting parental decision? Cureus 2021;9:11, e19415.
9. Simpson E, Carstensen J, Murphy P. Neonatal circumcision: new recommendations & implications for practice. Mo Med 2014;111(3):222–30. PMID: 25011345; PMCID: PMC6179567.
10. Alden KR. Nursing care of the newborn and family. In: Perry SE, Lowdermilk DL, Cashion K, et al, editors. Maternal child nursing care. 7th edition. St Louis: Elsevier; 2023. p. 565–8.
11. Taeusch HW, Martinez AM, Partridge JC, et al. Pain during mogen or plastibell circumcision. J Perinatol 2002;22:214–8.
12. Qahtani RA, Abu-Salem LY, Pal K. Effect of lidocaine-prilocaine eutectic mixture of local anaesthetic cream compared with oral sucrose or both in alleviating pain in neonatal circumcision procedure. Afr J Paediatr Surg 2014;11:1.
13. Raja SN, Carr DB, Cohen M, et al. The revised international association for the study of pain definition of pain: concepts, challenges, and compromises. Pain 2020;161:9. https://doi.org/10.1097/j.pain.0000000000001939.
14. Ricci SS, Kyle T, Carman S. Maternity and pediatric nursing. 4th edition592. Philadelphia: Wolters Kluwer; 2021. p. 1244–8.
15. American College of Obstetricians and Gynecologists, Facts are important: gestational development and capacity for pain, Available at: https://www.acog.org/advocacy/facts-are, 2024. Accessed February 25, 2024.

16. Oliveira IM, Castral TC, Cavalcante MMFP, et al. Nursing professionals' knowledge and attitude related to assessment and treatment of neonatal pain. Rev Eletr Enf 2016;18:e1160. Accessed February 13, 2024.

17. Dames LJP, Alves VH, Rodrigues DP, et al. Nurses' practical knowledge on the clinical management of neonatal pain: a descriptive study, *Online Brazil Journal of Nursing*, 15 (3), 2016, 393–403, Available at: http://www.objnursing.uff.br/index.php/nursing/article/view/5413. Accessed February 25, 2024.

18. Polkki T, Korhonen A, Laukkala H. Nurses' perceptions of pain assessment and management practices in neonates: a cross-sectional survey. Scand J Caring Sci 2018;32:725–33.

19. Garcia-Rodriguez MT, Bujan-Bravo S, Seijo-Bestilleiro R, et al. Pain assessment and management in the newborn: a systematized review. World Clin Cases 2021;21:5921–31.

20. Hellsten MB. Pain assessment in children. In: Hockenberry MJ, Duffy EA, Gibbs KD, editors. Wong's nursing care of infants and children. 12th edition. St. Louis: Elsevier; 2024. p. 139.

21. Stevens BJ, Gibbens S, Yamada J, et al. The premature infant pain profile-revised (PIPP-R): initial validation and feasibility. Clin J Pain 2014;30:238–43.

22. Lawrence J, Alcock D, McGrath P, et al. The development of a tool to assess neonatal pain. Neonatal Network: Nucleosides Nucleotides 1993;12(6):59–66.

23. Hummel P, Puchalski M, Creech SD, et al. Clinical reliability and validity of the N-PASS: neonatal pain, agitation, and sedation scale with prolonged pain. J Perinatol 2008;28(1):55–60.

24. van Dijk M, Roofthoot DWE, Anand KJS, et al. Taking up the challenge of measuring prolonged pain in (premeature)neotates: the COMFORTneo scale seems promising. Clin J Pain 2009;25(7):607–16.

25. Krechel SW, Bildner J. CRIES: A new neonatal postoperative pain measurement score. Initial testing of validity and reliability. Pediatric Anaesthesia 1995;5:53–61.

26. Razmus IS, Dalton ME, Wilson D. Pain management for newborn circumcision. Pediatr Nurs 2004;30(5):414–27.

27. Thacker JP, Shah DS, Patel DV, et al. Practices of procedural pain management in neonates through continuous quality improvement measures. Int J Pediatr 2022;7. Article ID 8605071.

28. Ogundele IO, Nwokoro CC, Adedeji TA, et al. Comparison of dorsal penile nerve block alone and in combination with lidocaine-prilocaine cream in neonates undergoing circumcision: a randomized controlled study. World Jnl Ped Surgery 2022;5:e000470.

29. Liu Y, Huang X, Luo B, et al. Effects of combined oral sucrose and nonnutritive sucking (NNS) on procedural pain of NICU newborns, 2001 to 2016: a PRISMA-compliant systematic review and meta-analysis. Medicine 2017;96(6):e6108.

30. Wang J, Zhao S, Luo L, et al. Dorsal penile nerve block versus eutectic mixture of local anesthetics cream for pain relief in infants during circumcision: a meta-analysis. PLoS One 2018;13(9):e0203439. Available at: https://doi.org/10.1371/journal.pone.0203439. Accessed February 25, 2024.

31. Stolik-Dollberg OC, Dollberg S. Bupivacaine versus lidocaine analgesia for neonatal circumcision. BMC Pediatr 2005;5:12. Available at: https://doi.org/10.1186/1471-2431-5-12. Accessed February 25, 2024.

32. Persad E, Pizzaro AB, Bruschettini M. Non-opioid analgesics for procedural pain in neonates. Cochrane Libr 2023. Available at: https://www.cochranelibrary.com/cdsr/doi/10.1002/14651858.CD015179.pub2/full. Accessed February 25, 2024.

33. Cregin R, Rappaport AS, Montagnino R, et al. Case study: Improving pain management for pediatric patients undergoing nonurgent painful procedures. Am J Health Syst Pharm 2008;65:723–7.

34. Taddio A, Pollock N, Gilbert-MacLeod C, et al. Combined analgesia and local anesthesia to minimize pain during circumcision. Arch Pediatr Adolesc Med 2000;154(6):620–3.

35. Qiaohong L, Xuerong T, Xueqing L, et al. Efficacy and safety of combined oral sucrose and nonnutritive sucking in pain management for infants: a systematic review and meta-analysis. PLoS One 2022. https://doi.org/10.1371/journal.pone.0268033.

36. McKinney ES, Murray SS, Mau K, et al. Maternal-child nursing. 6th edition. St. Louis: Elsevier; 2022. p. 479.

37. Vinall J, Grunau RE. Impact of repeated procedural pain-related stress in infants born very preterm. Pediatr Res 2014;75(5):584–7.

Strategies for Health Professionals in Managing Patients and Families in Critical Care Units

Mary Suzanne White, DNP, RN, PHCNS-BC,
Lynn C. Parsons, PhD, RN, NEA-BC*

KEYWORDS

- Pain • Stress • Burnout syndrome • Employee assistance programs
- Pain management certification

KEY POINTS

- Family knowledge can enhance quality of care at the bedside.
- Nurses lack pain management knowledge.
- Nurses experience work-related stress and burnout syndrome.
- Employee assistance programs offer interventions to manage work-related stress.

BACKGROUND

Health care professionals working in critical care units experience a difficult environment full of uncertainties. This environment becomes increasingly complex with the addition of multidisciplinary healthcare teams and ethical dilemmas associated with critical or end of life care.[1] Registered nurses (RNs), serving as pivotal figures in patient care, play a unique role as intermediaries between their hospitalized family members and the medical staff.[2,3] Evidenced-based practice underscores the importance of family involvement in hospital care and active participation in decision-making processes.[4] Notably, family expectations extend to being present during resuscitation efforts in cardiac arrest.[5,6] Critical care nurses, acting as patient advocates, can leverage family knowledge to enhance the quality of care at the bedside.

MANAGING STRESS IN THE CRITICAL CARE UNIT

Having a critically ill relative significantly affects families. Many families report grief, worry, despair, anxiety, and confusion which can lead to depression, insomnia, and

School of Health Sciences, Morehead State University, 201 Center for Health, Education and Research, 316 West Second Street, Morehead, KY 40351, USA
* Corresponding author.
E-mail address: Lynn.Parsons@mail.waldenu.edu

Crit Care Nurs Clin N Am 36 (2024) 531–538
https://doi.org/10.1016/j.cnc.2024.04.003
0899-5885/24/© 2024 Elsevier Inc. All rights reserved.

post-traumatic stress disorder.[7] Families of critical care patients describe their situations as complicated and deeply emotional experiences having physical, mental, and emotional impact. It is a tumultuous time accentuated by high *stress* levels and disruption to an entire family unit. Critical care nurses are instrumental in providing care for family members by providing information, comfort, support, and by acknowledging their presence as part of the critical care team.[8] Nurses having more experience or higher levels of education exhibit a deeper-rooted understanding of patient and family needs which may lead to better outcomes.[9]

Evidence-based practice related to critical care health care professionals' bedside interaction with patients' families from an ethical perspective has been studied and the following conclusions noted.[7]

- Quality care of families of critically ill patients depended on health care professionals' attitudes, behaviors, and personality traits.
- Attentive, active, and tolerant health care professionals symbolize a culture of ethics that encourages freedom and active participation of family members.
- Creating a culture of ethics for families must be established through education, interprofessional learning, and support of critical care health care professionals by health care facilities.[7]

PAIN MANAGEMENT IN CRITICAL CARE

Pain is complex and consists of sensory, emotional, and cognitive components. The sensory component relates to where a patient identifies pain in the body and how that pain is described. The emotional component includes feelings and affects associated with painful experiences. The cognitive component reflects how the patient attaches meaning to pain and can include expectations and past experiences. Because pain is highly subjective, self-report is the best assessment tool. Pain intensity is impossible to determine by any other means than self-report. Unfortunately, there are times when self-reporting pain is impossible and non-verbal signs of pain become more important.[10] These signs include:

- Facial expressions
- Vocalizations
- Body movements
- Altered interpersonal interactions
- Increase or decrease in activity
- Mental status change[10]

A significant responsibility of critical care nurses is to alleviate *pain* and provide comfort. This includes managing both acute and chronic pain associated with critical care procedures and routine interventions.[3] Unfortunately, there is a tendency among some RNs to under-assess, lack a full understanding, and under-treat pain. *Pain management*, a national concern and a substantial contributor to nurse stress in critical care units, is best addressed through a collaborative health professional team approach. Critical care nurses, being consistently at the bedside, play a crucial role in assessing, intervening, and relieving patient pain. Although research indicates nurses' knowledge and attitude toward pain management have a positive effect on reducing pain many RNs often lack current education on pain management.[11] Knowledge deficits and questionable attitudes among nurses pose obstacles to effective pain management. Also, many critical care nurses lack effective critical thinking and intuitive decision-making skills related to pain management. Negative nurse attitudes toward patient pain, inadequate pain assessment skills, misconceptions about patient behavior, and an overreliance on vital signs contribute to suboptimal pain management practices. Ineffective pain management is associated with longer hospital stays. Other negative outcomes include increased morbidity, mortality rates, and treatment costs.[12–14]

Concerns regarding the opioid epidemic can also contribute to pain undermanagement. Evidence-based research showcases the recent development of μ-receptor activity modulating opioids that are beneficial in pain management without typical adverse effects. This promotes a wider therapeutic window than traditional opioids.[12] Clinical studies indicate that oliceridine (TRV130), an innovative μ-receptor G-protein pathway-selective modulator, decreased postoperative pain with fewer adverse events when compared with morphine.[12]

Approaches to pain management of critical care patients should combine both pharmacologic and non-pharmacologic interventions. Non-pharmacologic interventions may enhance traditional pharmacologic interventions and may decrease the need for opioids.[15] Barriers to using non-pharmacological pain management methods among critical care RNs include fatigue, many responsibilities, heavy workload, and being understaffed. Nurses with higher levels of pain management knowledge and those holding bachelor's degrees are more likely to use non-pharmacological pain management methods than nurses with lower levels of knowledge or education.[16,17] Nurses must be well educated in pain relief methods, have the ability to assess method appropriateness for individual patients, and be able to deliver quality pain management.[18–20]

BURNOUT AMONG CRITICAL CARE HEALTH PROFESSIONALS

Critical care nurses experience work-related stressors associated with caring for high acuity patients requiring difficult or futile interventions and daily interaction with patient pain, trauma, and tragedy. Other reported work-related stressors include managing ethical dilemmas and increased clerical duties, including electronic medical record (EMR) documentation requirements.[21–23] While all health care professionals experience workplace stress, critical care nurses are at higher risk which can gradually lead to *burnout syndrome*. Burnout syndrome is defined as an individual's response to work-related stressors and is associated with negative consequences for health care professionals, patients, families, and the overall health care system. Sociodemographic factors such as being younger, single marital status, and having less professional experience in critical care influence the risk of burnout syndrome.[24,25]

Anuj and colleagues investigated burnout syndrome in health care professionals working in critical care units. Participants included 58 providers comprised of 26 physicians, 22 nurses, 6 respiratory therapists, 3 pharmacists, and 1 case manager. Results indicated that 10 participants (17.9%) described their burnout as moderate to high.[26] However, the following traits were reported among participants.

- 71.4% experienced emotional exhaustion
- 53.6% experienced depersonalization
- 53.6% experienced lack of personal achievement[26]

Burnout syndrome is related to high acuity patient care, team dynamics, and environmental culture. Individual factors included medical futility, difficult relationships with families, coworker burnout, lack of respect between team members, increasing administrative responsibilities, which decreased time for patient care, lack of recognition from administration and leadership, and technology.[26] Other evidence-based research related to workplace stress and burnout syndrome includes a study designed to investigate associations among critical care nurses' physical and mental health, perception of workplace wellness support, and self-reported medical errors. A total of 771 members of the American Association of Critical-Care Nurses participated in the study and the outcomes of interest included overall health, symptoms of depression and anxiety, stress, burnout, perceived worksite wellness support, and medical errors. Results indicated that critical care nurses in poor physical and mental health reported significantly more medical errors than nurses in better health and that nurses who perceived their worksite was very supportive of their well-being were twice as likely to have better physical health.[27] A third study aimed to explore whether fatigue, workload, burnout, and the work environment can predict the perceptions of patient safety among critical care nurses, determined a negative correlation between fatigue and patient safety culture. This indicates that nurse fatigue has a detrimental effect on perceptions of safety. There was also a significant relationship between work environment, emotional exhaustion, depersonalization, personal accomplishment, and facility patient safety culture.[28]

EMPLOYEE ASSISTANCE PROGRAMS FOR WORKLOAD STRESS MANAGEMENT

Many health care organizations are implementing *employee assistance programs* (EAPs) to better manage work-related stressors and prevent burnout syndrome among health care professionals. EAPs can include health care team approaches such as safe staffing ratios, alternating work schedules, recognition from administration and

---

Box 1
Case study – work-related stress

Samantha Snow is a RN who has practiced in the intensive care unit (ICU) for the past 5 years. Before this appointment, she practiced on acute medical-surgical units for 9 years. She has weathered changes over the past 14 years and finds herself stressed because she has heavy patient loads with high acuity levels requiring extensive care. Most of the ICU patients experience acute and chronic pain and encounter pain during care procedures. She is further stressed by the family who visits often. The hospital policy supports family visitation for 10 minutes every hour between 9:00 AM and 8:00 PM each day.

Samantha is a charge nurse often for her 7:00 AM – 7:30 PM shift. She is a full-time employee that works 7 shifts every 2 weeks. She holds a BSN degree and reports that her major education relative to pain management was in nursing school 14 years ago. She reports feeling burned out and stressed at work for the past few months. Other nurses are experiencing this same phenomenon.

She has voiced that family presence on the unit contributes to her stress. Samantha is reported to be a team-player, is clinically proficient, helps other staff with their patient care assignments and is a good leader. She is highly respected by staff nurse colleagues, the interdisciplinary team and members of the medical staff.

Discussion Questions
1. What can upper-level supervisors, including the chief nursing officer (CNO) to alleviate Samantha's job stress?
2. What interventions can upper-level supervisors, including the chief nursing officer (CNO), do to enhance/increase pain management knowledge, including nursing interventions for the ICU nursing staff?
3. Should the ICU policy for family visitation be reviewed? What potential changes to the policy may benefit patients, families, and the interdisciplinary team? If it is determined that changes should be made, who should be included in policy revision?

See **Box 2** for answers to these questions.

Box 2
Case study – work-related stress

Responses to Discussion Questions

1. What can upper-level supervisors, including the chief nursing officer (CNO) to alleviate Samantha's job stress?
   - Rotate the Charge Nurse role among the other, experienced ICU nursing staff. This strategy will increase nurse leader skills among many qualified staff RNs and equally distribute a comprehensive practice role.
   - Provide a schedule for lunch or 15-min breaks. Seasoned nursing supervisors could assist in providing coverage as competent, qualified staffing is often an issue in ICU settings.
   - Offer flexible work schedules.
   - Assure safe nurse to staff patient ratios.
   - Offer employee assistance programs to prevent and/or manage stress. Types of programs may include:
     ○ Offer yoga sessions.
     ○ Provide gym passes.
     ○ Provide mental health resources.
     ○ Have stress management workshops.
     ○ Mindfulness programs – Meditation, Body Scan Exercise (body awareness) - Retrieved from: https://www.mayoclinic.org/healthy-lifestyle/consumer-health/in-depth/mindfulness-exercises/art-20046356#:~:text=Mindfulness%20is%20a%20type%20of,mind%20and%20help%20reduce%20stress.

2. What interventions can upper-level supervisors, including the chief nursing officer (CNO), do to enhance/increase pain management knowledge, including nursing interventions for the ICU nursing staff?
   - Review the rules and regulations of the state Board of Nursing. Some state regulators require continuing education hours on the topic of pain and pain management. State Boards of Nursing frequently offer continuing education units (CEU) on different topics. They also recommend CEU courses on several topics, including pain.
   - Offer staff development sessions on pain management. Consider hiring a Pain Clinical Nurse Specialist with extensive knowledge in acute and chronic pain management.
   - Fiscally support ICU RNs in attending pain management conferences and workshops.
   - Support hospital libraries in securing refereed nursing journals focusing on critical care, acute and chronic pain management and pain assessment and intervention practice skills.
   - Support RNs in obtaining certification in pain management. The American Nurses Credentialing Center (ANCC) offers a *Pain Management Nursing Certification* (PMGT-BC). Eligibility requirements to take the certification exam are:
     ○ Current, active RN license in the United States, its territories, or Canada. A minimum of 2 years of full-time practice as an RN.
     ○ A minimum number of hours of pain management nursing experience and completing relevant continuing education. Retrieved from: https://www.linkedin.com/pulse/ancc-pmgt-bc-exam-pain-management-nursing-certification?trk=article-ssr-frontend-pulse_more-articles_related-content-card

3. Should the ICU policy for family visitation be reviewed? What potential changes to the policy may benefit patients, families, and the interdisciplinary team? If it is determined that changes should be made, who should be included in policy revision?
   Yes, ICU visitation policies should be reviewed.
   - Review the literature for current, evidence-based ICU visitor policies.
   - Survey other hospital organizations to determine how they manage ICU visitation. Ask what types of issues they may have and how they are managed.
   - Invite diverse people to review, edit and finalize ICU visitor policies. Suggestions include:
     ○ Hospital chaplain or ethicist
     ○ Nurses in acute, critical, or mental health units
     ○ Community Leaders
     ○ Members of the healthcare interdisciplinary team, including physicians
     ○ Nurse administrator(s), including the Chief Nursing Officer (CNO)

leadership, and team building. Additionally, EAPs can offer education tailored to critical care RNs including pain management and the role of family in patient care and decision making. Individual employee initiatives include self-care stress management and relaxation techniques training, and self-care health education opportunities such as nutrition, exercise, meditation, and sleep hygiene measures.[21,29,30] A 2020 systematic review of studies published between 2009 to 2019 targeting management of work-related stressors experienced by critical care health care professionals was conducted.[31] Findings included the consensus that cognitive-behavioral skills training and mindfulness-based interventions are effective in managing work-related stressors among critical care health care professionals, including nurses.[31] Additionally, there is mounting evidence that the role of positive emotion is effective in managing work-related stress and avoiding burnout syndrome. By providing individuals with positive emotion skill building interventions, critical care healthcare professionals can learn to be in the moment through formal or informal measures, to better appreciate the work environment and celebrate patient achievement.[21]

Although there is a plethora of research on critical care work-related stress and interventions for management, it is not clear if they are of appropriate methodological quality. This article highlights the need for high methodological quality studies to ensure recommended interventions are truly evidence based.[31]

SUMMARY

Critical care nurses in intensive care unit settings shoulder numerous responsibilities, including the management of complex health issues compounded by acute and chronic pain. Critical care nurses should enhance knowledge regarding pain and pain management methods, including opioids that can enhance patient comfort. Attitudes toward pain should also be investigated. Improved knowledge and attitude regarding pain management can result in higher patient and family satisfaction, as well as high quality and safe outcomes.[32] Critical care nurses suffer from emotional exhaustion and often have risk factors for burnout syndrome including being younger, single marital status, and having less professional experience in critical care units. Other work-related factors include workload and long hours.[25] Recognizing the stressful nature of the critical care environment, it is imperative that hospital leaders provide adequate support to critical care nurses. There is a need for high methodological quality studies to ascertain such programs are evidence-based. Refer to **Boxes 1** and **2** for a case study addressing stress management for a critical care nurse.

CLINICS CARE POINTS

- Critical care nurses play a crucial role in assessing, intervening, and relieving patient pain.
- Critical care health care professionals experience higher rates of mental distress and poor health, which negatively affects the quality of patient and family care.
- Health care leaders and systems should make the health of professionals a priority by addressing identified system issues, promoting wellness environments, and implementing evidence-based interventions.

DISCLOSURE

All authors report no commercial or financial conflicts of interest. There was no funding from any source for this publication.

REFERENCES

1. Othman SY, Hassan NI, Mohamed AM. Effectiveness of mindfulness-based interventions on burnout and self-compassion among critical care nurses caring for patients with COVID-19: a quasi-experimental study. BMC Nurs 2023;22(1):305.

2. Deek H, Hamilton S, Brown N, et al. Family-centred approaches to healthcare interventions in chronic diseases in adults: a quantitative systematic review. J Adv Nurs 2016;72(5):968–79.

3. Park M, Giap TT, Lee M, et al. Patient- and family-centered care interventions for improving the quality of health care: a review of systematic reviews. Int J Nurs Stud 2018;87:69–83.

4. Kokorelias KM, Gignac MAM, Naglie G, et al. Towards a universal model of family centered care: a scoping review. BMC Health Serv Res 2019;19(1):564.

5. Douma MJ, Graham TAD, Ali S, et al. What are the care needs of families experiencing cardiac arrest?: a survivor and family led scoping review. Resuscitation 2021;168:119–41.

6. Cornell R, Powers K. Advancing the practice of family presence during resuscitation: a multifaceted hospital-wide interprofessional program. Dimens Crit Care Nurs 2022;41(6):286–94.

7. Nygaard AM, Haugdahl HS, Laholt H, et al. Professionals' narratives of interactions with patients' families in intensive care. Nurs Ethics 2022;29(4):885–98.

8. McAndrew NS, Schiffman R, Leske J. A theoretical lens through which to view the facilitators and disruptors of nurse-promoted engagement with families in the ICU. J Fam Nurs 2020;26(3):190–212.

9. Kynoch K, Ramis MA, McArdle A. Experiences and needs of families with a relative admitted to an adult intensive care unit: a systematic review of qualitative studies. JBI Evid Synth 2021;19(7):1499–554.

10. Sampson EL, West E, Fischer T. Pain and delirium: mechanisms, assessment, and management. Eur Geriatr Med 2020;11(1):45–52.

11. Samarkandi OA. Knowledge and attitudes of nurses toward pain management. Saudi J Anaesth 2018;12(2):220–6.

12. Gan TJ. Poorly controlled postoperative pain: prevalence, consequences, and prevention. J Pain Res 2017;10:2287–98.

13. Joshi GP, Kehlet H. Postoperative pain management in the era of ERAS: an overview. Best Pract Res Clin Anaesthesiol 2019;33(3):259–67.

14. van Boekel RLM, Warlé MC, Nielen RGC, et al. Relationship between postoperative pain and overall 30-day complications in a broad surgical population: an observational study. Ann Surg 2019;269(5):856–65.

15. Sandvik RK, Olsen BF, Rygh LJ, et al. Pain relief from nonpharmacological interventions in the intensive care unit: a scoping review. J Clin Nurs 2020;29(9–10):1488–98.

16. Ocak C, Yildizeli ST. The role of nurses' knowledge and attitudes in postoperative pain management. Colegn 2023;30(56):715–20.

17. Zeinab K, Allahbakhshian M, Ilkhani M, et al. Nurses' use of non-pharmacological pain management methods in intensive care units: a descriptive cross-sectional study. Compl Ther Med 2021;58:102705.

18. Mahama F, Ninnoni JPK. Assessment and management of postoperative pain among nurses at a resource-constraint teaching hospital in Ghana. Nurs Res Pract 2019;2019:9091467.

19. Meissner W, Huygen F, Neugebauer EAM, et al. Management of acute pain in the postoperative setting: the importance of quality indicators. Curr Med Res Opin 2018;34(1):187–96.
20. Rababa M, Al-Rawashdeh S. Critical care nurses' critical thinking and decision making related to pain management. Intensive Crit Care Nurs 2021;63:103000.
21. Cheung EO, Hernandez A, Herold E, et al. Positive emotion skills intervention to address burnout in critical care nurses. AACN Adv Crit Care 2020;31(2):167–78.
22. Kane L. Medscape National physician burnout and depression report. 2019. Available at: https://www.medscape.com/slideshow/2019-lifestyle-burnout-depression-6011056/.
23. Wright AA, Katz IT. Beyond burnout - redesigning care to restore meaning and sanity for physicians. N Engl J Med 2018;378(4):309–11.
24. Moss M, Good VS, Gozal D, et al. A Critical Care Societies collaborative statement: burnout syndrome in critical care health-care professionals: a call for action. Am J Respir Crit Care Med 2016;194:106–13.
25. Ramírez-Elvira S, Romero-Béjar JL, Suleiman-Martos N, et al. Prevalence, risk factors and burnout levels in intensive care unit nurses: a systematic review and meta-analysis. Int J Environ Res Publ Health 2021;18(21):11432.
26. Mehta AB, Lockhart S, Reed K, et al. Drivers of burnout among critical care providers: a multicenter mixed-methods study. Chest 2022;161(5):1263–74.
27. Melnyk BM, Tan A, Hsieh AP, et al. Critical care nurses' physical and mental health, worksite wellness support, and medical errors. Am J Crit Care 2021;30(3):176–84.
28. Al Ma'mari Q, Sharour LA, Al Omari O. Fatigue, burnout, work environment, workload and perceived patient safety culture among critical care nurses. Br J Nurs 2020;29(1):28–34.
29. West CP, Dyrbye LN, Erwin PJ, et al. Interventions to prevent and reduce physician burnout: a systematic review and meta-analysis. Lancet 2016;388(10057):2272–81.
30. Panagioti M, Panagopoulou E, Bower P, et al. Controlled interventions to reduce burnout in physicians: a systematic review and meta-analysis. JAMA Intern Med 2017;177(2):195–205.
31. Alkhawaldeh JMA, Soh KL, Mukhtar FBM, et al. Stress management interventions for intensive and critical care nurses: a systematic review. Nurs Crit Care 2020;25(2):84–92.
32. Brant JM, Mohr C, Coombs NC, et al. Nurses' knowledge and attitudes about pain: personal and professional characteristics and patient reported pain satisfaction. Pain Manag Nurs 2017;18(4):214–23.

Guided Imagery and Other Complementary Pain Control Approaches for Critical Care Patients

Jenny Pappas, DNP, APRN, FNP-C[a], Lori A. Sutton, MSN, RN[a],
Debra Rose Wilson, PhD, MSN, RN, IBCLC, AHN-BC, CHT[b],*

KEYWORDS

- Complementary • Pain management • Non-opioid approaches • ICU patients
- Ventilator patients • Pain

KEY POINTS

- Numerous assessment tools are available for critical nurses to assess the levels of pain, anxiety, and delirium in ICU patients.
- Using complementary approaches to address anxiety and pain in ICU-ventilated patients reduces hospital stays.
- Sedation and pain medication can be reduced with complementary therapies that nurses and the interdisciplinary ICU team can implement.

Background

Pain is one of the most common ailments critical care nurses tend to daily. Annually, over 5 million patients are admitted to the critical care unit, with over half of these patients experiencing pain at rest and approximately 80% experiencing acute pain with procedures.[1] Undiagnosed and unmanaged pain for this population directly impacts the patient's health, rest, oxygen consumption, and immune function and increases the likelihood of dementia and trauma.[1,2] Patients may come to the intensive care unit (ICU) with previously diagnosed pain or experience procedural or acute pain from their current diagnosis.

The critical care patient is often unable to verbalize pain, making it imperative to use evidence-based pain assessment tools to identify pain in patients. These tools are for both ventilated and nonverbal patients. Appropriate pain assessment and management

[a] Austin Peay State University, 601 College Street, Clarksville, TN 37044, USA; [b] Austin Peay State University, Walden University, 601 College Street, Clarksville, TN 37044, USA
* Corresponding author.
E-mail address: debrarosewilson@comcast.net

in critical care patients result in improved outcomes, including shorter length of stay, less incidence of delirium, and lower mortality rates (**Box 1**).[1–3]

Pain Assessment

There are a variety of pain assessments used in intensive care settings. Self-reported or subjective pain scales are the most reliable method and should be the first choice if the patient can respond.[1] The most common self-reported pain scales in acute care settings include a numeric scale rating (0–10) and the provocation, quality, region (or radiation), severity (or scale), and timing (PQRST) mnemonic. The PQRST mnemonic includes assessing what provokes/palliates the pain, the quality/quantity of the pain, the region/radiation of the pain, the severity of the pain, and the timing of the pain.[4] When patients cannot self-report pain, other validated, objective tools can be used.

The 2 most common pain scales used in the ICU include the Critical Care Pain Observation Tool (CPOT) and the Behavioral Pain Scale (BPS). These pain scales scored the highest psychometric through their research.[4] The CPOT assesses facial expressions, body movements, compliance with mechanical ventilation, and muscle tension. The scoring system for CPOT is 0 (no pain) to 8 (maximum pain); intervention is recommended starting at a score of 2. This tool has scored excellent inter-rater reliability (k = 0.62–0.88), with its validity and reliability confirmed, though it is most effective for non-agitated patients.[4] This tool can be found by downloading the .pdf at this link.

The BPS assesses 3 categories: facial expression, upper limb movement, and compliance with mechanical ventilation. Behavioral pain scores range from 4 (no pain) to 12 (maximum pain). The BPS scale recommends intervention starting for pain at a score of 6.[1] Both the CPOT and the BPS tools are available at www.ncbi.nlm.nih.gov/pmc/articles/PMC6390431/ and are recognized as the most commonly used tools.[5]

PHARMACOLOGIC AND NONPHARMACOLOGIC APPROACHES TO PAIN MANAGEMENT

Pharmacologic pain management in critical care patients has been the practice standard. The side effects and the long-term risks of pharmacologic pain management, specifically opioid use, are now considered. Opioid overdose is now the third leading cause of death in the United States, with the incidence growing 400% since 1999 and another 30% since 2020.[6] Opioid use can also increase patient risk for delirium. While opioids and other pharmacologic pain medications are an essential part of pain management for many critical care patients, a multi-modal approach, including nonpharmacologic approaches, has the highest quality outcomes for the patient.

The lowest dose of sedation and analgesia is used in ventilated and other ICU patients to address comfort but ensure safety. This approach reduces oxygen demand and excessive sedation but has been shown to prolong ventilation, increase cost, and

---

Box 1
Acute vs. Chronic Pain

Acute pain is defined as short-term (less than 6 months), self-limiting, and resolving after the injury heals. Chronic pain lasts 6 months or longer and typically does not stop when the injury heals.[3]

reduce patient outcomes.[2] Beyond opioids, and even beyond over-the-counter anti-inflammatories and other painkillers, there are numerous evidence-based approaches to both acute and chronic pain. Pain is a leading stressor among ICU patients and may not be related to their current condition.[7] There are numerous complementary and evidenced-based approaches to pain management that might be suggested and implemented by the nurse caring for critical care patients with pain.

GUIDED IMAGERY AND HYPNOSIS

Guided imagery is a nurse-initiated tool to help patients do more than just relax. The physiologic benefits include positive changes in heart rate, blood pressure, pain levels, anxiety levels, and immune function. Imagery was used in ancient Greece and in traditional Chinese Medicine, American Indian, and Australian Aboriginal people.[8] Guided imagery is classified as a mind-body technique that uses detailed mental images and is like telling a story. The brain is guided to visualize an experience in a positive, affirming, and comforting way. The goal should be clearly stated in the beginning. The process involves all 5 senses and transports the patient to a safe and peaceful place. In a trance-like state, the mind is more accepting of positive affirmations.[6] The imagination can be used to override physiologic function. Visualizing using all 5 senses in the story has enormous power in making positive changes in biology and function.[8]

Guided imagery is recognized as an effective relaxation technique for adult ICU patients, and it is recommended in clinical guidelines for adult ICU patients.[4] The use of guided imagery can induce relaxation or even sleep. Sleep in the ICU is often impaired or fragmented, and a lack of deep or rapid eye movement (REM) stages of sleep impairs immune function and increases the incidence of ICU delirium.[4] There are no adverse effects. Guided imagery can be used for most populations, though it should be avoided when the patients are experiencing delusions, hallucinations, or psychosis, as the experience may complicate their understanding of reality.[6]

Guided imagery is passive, where the patient listens to the nurse (or an audio tape) and focuses on pleasant images. The experience of the senses (what the patient would feel, hear, see, taste, and smell) in that situation is reinforced to help create the image in the conscious and subconscious areas of cognition. There is research supporting its use on pain and anxiety and impacting the use of restraint in ICU.[9] A 2021 study[10] found that guided imagery had a positive effect on anxiety, muscle pain, and vital signs for patients with COVID-19. The pain intensity was reduced, and the quality of the pain was moderated. Oxygen saturation and blood pressure all indicated further relaxation effects of the guided imagery.[10]

When using guided imagery, it is important to find a "place" where there is peace and safety for each patient. A beach scene may be relaxing for most, but there will be the patient who experienced a shark bite or witnessed a near drowning, and the scene elicits anxiety.

There is research supporting the use of guided imagery specific to ICU patients, but more research is needed. The physiologic framework (**Fig. 1**) applies to the ICU patient and helps illustrate how guided imagery works. Guided imagery has no significant risk and can be employed during or before a procedure to reduce pain, induce relaxation, and help sleep (**Box 2**). Future research needs to focus on the improvement of critically ill patients specific to guided imagery. Double-blind procedures are needed to minimize bias, and statistical analysis needs to examine the effect of guided imagery over time.[11]

Hypnosis is a deeper trance-like state and is more interactive between the hypnotherapist and the patient. Hypnosis often begins with a guided imagery. Hypnosis

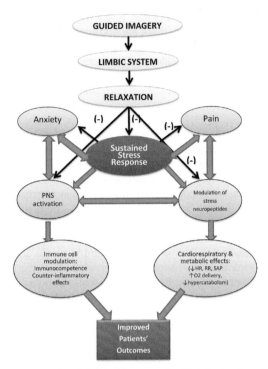

Fig. 1. Physiologic Framework of Guided Imagery by Hadjibalassi and colleagues (2018). (Rights requested January 2, 2024, from Elsevier.)

provides opportunities for personal growth and insight and is effective in pain management but does require the patient to respond cognitively and verbally. The Clinical Practice Guidelines on managing pain and delirium in adult ICU patients do not recognize hypnosis as an appropriate intervention for the very ill ICU patients because of a

---

Box 2
Example of a guided imagery script for sleep based on a disclosure of a positive childhood memory

Take a breath in and take a moment to settle yourself. As you breathe out, focus on relaxing the muscles of your jaw and shoulders. Take another breath and soften the muscles of your jaw and shoulders again. You are in a safe place. One more breath.

Imagine yourself back in your grandmother's kitchen. You are between 4 and 6 years old and sitting at the table watching your grandmother make cookies. The smell of sweet vanilla and chocolate fills the air. The dishes are washed and carefully stacked to dry by the white porcelain sink. The sound of water running and dishes tinkling is comforting. The taste of warm cocoa fills your mouth as you sip on the cup that Grandma made for each of you. The sound of a gentle wind through the oak trees outside makes a rustle and the leaves of fall are beginning to descend. Grandma comes over with the cookies, still warm and gooey on a plate. One for each of you. You and Grandma make a great ceremony of dipping the warm cookie into the cocoa. Grandma's warm and loving arm is around you as you breathe into this moment of quiet and stillness. You feel drowsy and peaceful; you are loved. All is right for this moment in time. You can rest.

lack of solid clinical studies.[4] Critical care nurses can become certified in both guided imagery and clinical hypnosis and may find these tools valuable options for their patients and may inspire clinical research at the institution.

Guided imagery and hypnosis use relaxation and visualization to guide the patient into a trance-like state where the brain produces alpha waves. Hypnosis goes further and produces alpha and the slower, deeper theta waves.[6] A systematic review and meta-analysis (85 controlled experimental trials, with N = 3632) indicated that hypnosis provided moderate to large analgesia for all pain types.[12] The pain was significantly lowered with hypnosis in 64 of those studies. Forty-two percent of the participants reported optimal pain relief, and 29% reported clinically meaningful pain reduction. Hypnosis was found to be a safe and effective alternative to medication.[12]

ACUPUNCTURE

The efficiency of acupuncture, a 2000-year-old Chinese Medicine practice, is well established in the literature and recommended by the World Health Organization (WHO)[13] since 1979. The WHO now recommends acupuncture for over 100 conditions, including nausea, low back pain, hyper and hypotension, dysmenorrhea, addiction, and allergies. Acupuncture, however, is seldom used for the ICU-ventilated population. Acupuncture is an evidence-based technique that is thought to activate the flow of energy through the body that relieves pain, numbness, and heaviness.[14] While we do not, in a Western medicine mindset, understand how acupuncture works, it has been shown that mast cells, blood vessels, and nerve fibers mediate the signals from the inserted needles. Kinase (an enzyme) pathways are activated, causing a cascade of cell signaling and protein responses. Multiple transmitters and modulators, including endogenous opioids, cholecystokinin octapeptide, 5-hydroxytryptamine, noradrenaline, and dopamine, have been shown to be involved in acupuncture analgesia.[14] We do not clearly understand how acupuncture works, but researchers are beginning to understand how this ancient practice changes cellular and immune function at a quantum level.[6]

Zhang and colleagues[2] conducted a randomized trial on ICU ventilated patients using a control group (who received superficial acupuncture needle insertion at nonacupoints) and a non-treatment group who received no acupuncture or needles. Participants were randomized and those receiving the acupuncture treatment had the commonly used electrical stimulation bursts added to the needle during treatment. Pain, agitation, and sedation levels were measured using the Richmond Agitation Sedation Scale (RASS), the BPS, and Numeric Rating Scale. Delerium was measured by the Confusion Assessment Method (CAM) for ICU. Caregivers monitored for adverse effects and patients were monitored and care adjusted as per usual. Preliminary data published from this ongoing study reported that the group who had acupuncture reported less pain, like similar earlier studies of this population. The use of acupuncture is meaningful analgesia for patients in ICU.[2]

A groundbreaking retrospective study examining the experience of acupuncture for 73,406 patients found that around 7% of patients will have adverse effects that most commonly include site bleeding or bruising.[15] Significantly rarer but still a risk is infection from non-sterile needles or a nerve injury from a misplaced needle.[15] A meta-analysis published in 2023 found that critically ill patients in ICU who received acupuncture treatment had reduced time in the ICU, a lower 28-day mortality rate, and were found to have had no harm caused because of the intervention.[16] While minor adverse effects (bruising, bleeding) were noted 9.31% of the time, more serious side effects occur in about 1 in a million treatments.[16] Acupuncture might be a safe approach for a ventilated patient with current or chronic pain and may reduce the trauma of the ventilation experience.

Acupuncture is performed by someone certified in the techniques and this is monitored by the state or provincial health licensing board. Certifications for specific approaches in acupuncture are available for nurses. For example, nurses can become certified in auricular acupuncture (only in the pinna of the ear) used for addiction, chronic pain, anxiety, allergies, and weight loss where needles and seeds stimulate specific acupuncture sites.

MUSIC AND SOUND

The stress of the experience of being a ventilated ICU patient has been found to be reduced with music and sound therapy. The lit, loud, and active environment of an ICU has been known to add to the stress and agitation of patients. Music or sound-canceling headphones can be added to pharmaceutical approaches to manage pain, restlessness, anxiety, and delirium. Music and peaceful sounds tend to be soothing, though the personal choice in what is playing is relevant. Music is recommended as an approach to managing pain and delirium in adult ICU patients.[4]

A 2021 study examined the effect of music on delirium, sedation, anxiety, and pain in ventilated ICU patients.[17] They used ear plugs to provide music therapy and collected data on delirium (CAM for ICU), pain (CPOT), sedation (RASS), and anxiety (Facial Anxiety Scale). Music therapy had an anxiolytic effect, reducing the need for pharmaceutical sedation. The severity of pain and delirium were also noted with those who had music.[17]

Music therapy has also been studied during the weaning off a ventilator. While analgesics or sedatives are often used to reduce distress in the weaning experience, adding music may reduce the need for pharmaceuticals that often directly impair respiratory effort. Ventilated patients being weaned were (N = 30) divided randomly into 2 groups: one who had music therapy with weaning and one who had standard care.[18] Music therapy reduced pain and anxiety during the experience of weaning off the ventilator and recommended it as a safe, effective, and inexpensive intervention during extubation.[18]

COLD THERAPY

The clinical practice guidelines for prevention and management of pain and delirium in ICU patients recommend cold therapy for patient care protocols such as during chest tube removal based on earlier studies.[4] A 2018 study[19] conducted a study on 87 patients having chest tubes removed. Chest tube insertion and removal is a painful and traumatic experience. Cold application before the tube removal reduced the amount of pain reported during the intervention. The authors explained that application of cold slows tissue metabolism, slows neuron transfer, and has anti-inflammatory and analgesic properties.[19] Reported pain levels between the intervention and non-intervention groups were similar again after 15 minutes, telling us that cold therapy is a temporary approach and would be most effective for short-term procedural pain.[19]

PHYSICAL AND OCCUPATIONAL THERAPY AND MOVEMENT

There is a clear role for physical and occupational therapists in ventilated ICU patients. A large (N = 541) cohort 2020 study supported the practice of early mobilization for patients on mechanical ventilation.[20] They studied the effect of interdisciplinary proto-cols for MDs, nurses, PT, OT, and RT health professionals. This resulted in a change of protocols that decreased patient hospital days, decreased mortality, and improved physical function of the patient at discharge. A meta-analysis examined 60 clinical tri-als (N = 5352) and found that physical/occupational rehabilitation consistently improved function and reduced the length of hospital stay.[21] Other variables such as duration of ventilation, mortality, and quality of life were not statistically significant.

Pulmonary rehabilitation includes regular clearing of secretions with suction, vibra-tion, and percussion to reduce the work of breathing. Focusing on improving lung function enhances inflation, normalized chest movement, and respiratory muscle functioning, and restores normal lung function.[22] Positioning and mobilization assist with oxygenation and reduce long-term lung damage. Lung functional residual capac-ity and oxygenation improve when the patient is brought up to a more seated posi-tioning of greater than 30°.[23] Early mobilization or movement does have limitations for patients because of potential polytrauma, older chronic pain issues, or sudden forced immobility leading to ICU-acquired weakness.[22] However, a multidisciplinary approach to mobilization improves patient outcomes by reducing days in hospitals and improving long-term mobility.

MASSAGE

Massage therapy for ventilated ICU patients usually involves massage of the back, feet, or hands, and sometimes the abdomen. Massage is more effective when paired with dimmed lights and muting of audible alarms. The patient may benefit from an eye mask and either noise canceling headphones or ear plugs or soft music playing.[22] Massage is considered an appropriate intervention according to Clinical Practice Guidelines.[4]

Shiatsu massage is a complementary approach to healing that is used worldwide and based within traditional medical practices and massage of acupuncture points. It is a deep massage known to relieve pain and anxiety and enhance comfort and sleep.[24] Shiatsu massage was found to reduce agitation in (N = 68) ventilated pa-tients, reducing the need for pharmaceuticals. The researchers included patients who were 30 to 60 years of age, had a score of greater than 7 on the Glasgow Coma scale, and had agitation behaviors as determined by the RASS.[24] Two groups were studied, including a control group. Prior to the Shiatsu massage intervention, agitation scores between the control group (normal care protocols) and the interven-tion group were compared. After the massage, the intervention groups' agitation score decreased significantly when compared to the control group.[24] Shiatsu massage is effective in reducing agitation in ventilated ICU patients, though more studies are needed.

Current research for patients in the ICU continues to support the use of foot mas-sage. Except in rare cases, massage of the extremities is safe, relaxing, and will reduce the experience of pain for ICU patients.[25] ICU patients who received foot mas-sage therapy experienced decreased heart rate and respirations, and increased O_2 saturation (**Fig. 2**). Foot massage can be a safe, evidence-based way to improve the experience of being a ventilated patient in ICU.[25]

THE FAMILY'S EXPERIENCE

Having a family member hospitalized in the ICU is distressing. Family members of ICU patients report experiencing uncertainty, lack of communication with the health care team, and inflexibility with visiting policies as stressors. Witnessing their loved one

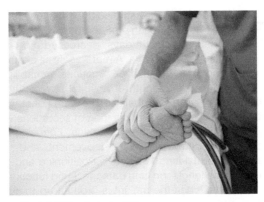

Fig. 2. Foot massage. (Sudok1/iStockphoto LP)

in pain can be traumatizing. Families experience disruption in their daily routines, conflict with roles, and adverse psychological effects.[26] Anxiety, depression, and post-traumatic stress disorder (PTSD) have been reported in up to 70% of family members.[26,27] During the hospitalization of their loved one, families report anxiety (42%–79.7%), depression (16% –90%), and PTSD (33%–82%).[26] Family members report continued strain and adverse effects on their mental health after discharge. At 6 months post-discharge, family members have reported anxiety (15%–24%) and depression (4.7%–36.4%).[26] Symptoms of PTSD have been reported (31.7%–80%) to continue into the year following discharge.[26]

SUPPORTING FAMILY MEMBERS

Witnessing a family member in pain because of their condition or a procedure is distressing and can be disturbing. A 2022 study[28] reported that the most stressful aspects of having a family member in the ICU was:

- A lack of information regarding their family member's treatment,
- Seeing the family member in pain,
- Uncertainty regarding treatment success,
- And fear of death.

Xyrichis[29] systematically reviewed the literature to identify interventions to promote adaptive coping and family member involvement in critical care units. After performing a comprehensive review of the literature, the researchers suggest that there is not a 'one size fits all' intervention to assist family members of ICU patients in adaptive coping; instead, they suggest nurses and health care team members 'screen and treat' family members individually.[29] The authors organized interventions into categories including cost, family involvement required, health care team involvement required, and outcome for the patient. Participation in medical rounds is a high commitment of family time that results in a high impact on communication at a meager cost but a very low impact on patient outcomes. Whereas multicomponent support, which utilized more than one technique to educate the family, resulted in a high commitment of family time and high cost with a moderate impact on patient outcomes with managing pain as an example. Utilizing this typology allows critical care nurses and health care team members to tailor the intervention based on their ICU setting.[29] Critical care nurses can utilize the family for history of pre-existing pain, and involve family in care, including complementary approaches for managing pain, confusion, and anxiety. Offering other approaches to managing the care of the patient provides another opportunity for family education and establishment of rapport.

ASSESSMENT TOOLS FOR FAMILIES OF THE INTENSIVE CARE UNIT PATIENT

Family of a ventilated patient has experienced an incidental crisis, an event that was caused by an unpredictable event.[30] The crisis continues until all members adapt to changes and new conditions and restore balance and stability.[30] During the crisis, the Family Crisis Oriented Evaluation Scales (F-COPES) can be utilized to assess the ways of coping among the family members.[30] The purpose of the scale is to identify and measure behavioral strategies used by families in response to problematic or difficult situations, such as patient agitation, pain, or confusion. The 30-item questionnaire surveys 5 strategies: seeking social support, the meaning of the situation, seeking out spiritual support, seeking outside help, and passive assessment of the situation. Critical care nurses can utilize the scale to assess family members' internal and external coping support.

The facilitated sensemaking model (FSM) provides critical care nurses with interventions that can prevent adverse psychological effects such as anxiety, depression, and PTSD in family members of ICU patients.[27] The model is based on 2 concepts. One, what is happening in the ICU, and two, how do I adapt to the new role of ICU caregiver? The FSM is arranged into 4 areas: caring relationships, communication, presence, and decision-making. An example of a caring relationship is incorporating the family members and respecting their input as part of the team when addressing pain or anxiety in the patient. Communication can be better achieved by discussing and reviewing met and unmet needs with the family. Presence can be exemplified by welcoming the family's presence at the bedside and involving them in caring and gentle approaches to managing pain. Decision-making can be reinforced by encouraging family discussion. Utilization of the FSM with family members of patients ventilated in the ICU reduced reported anxiety, depression, and PTSD. Evidence recommends that critical care nurses utilize a variety of interventions tailored to the family's and the patient's needs.[27]

The Family Satisfaction in the Intensive Care Unit-24 (FS ICU-24) is a validated tool to measure the family's satisfaction when a loved one is in the ICU.[31] The tool measures areas including patient care, family care, the ICU environment, and assessment of the decision-making process.[31] A 2021 study found that the items related to pain on the questionnaire received the highest satisfaction scores when pain was well addressed by nurses.[32]

Family-centered care (FCC) focuses on the needs and values of the family unit, of which the patient is a member (**Box 3**).[33] Finding ways to include families in patient care, especially complementary and compassionate approaches to pain management, are opportunities to educate and inform. Family members often feel empowered.

POST-CRITICAL CARE PATIENT CARE

Long-term hospitalization and possible mechanical ventilation have a lasting effect on a patient's mental, cognitive, and physical health. Post-Intensive Care Syndrome (PICS) is a term used to describe the psychological, physical, and cognitive impairments patients face after being discharged from the ICU.[34] The assessment, prevention, and treatment of pain are fundamental to reducing the frequency and severity of PICS. PICS was present long-term, with 60% of patients having it 1-month post-

---

Box 3
Schwartz[33] shared 5 best practices for FCC in the ICU

1. Encourage and facilitate family presence. Review strict visitation policies and use restrictions only when necessary.

2. Form empathetic, supporting, and friendly interactions with family.

3. Prioritize communication. Communicate regularly with honest, timely, transparent information, offering education and opportunity for questions.

4. Seek consultation. Consult with the OT and PT professionals, local acupuncturists, and pastoral or other spiritual support. Bring in patient massage therapists to provide services and teach the critical care nurses.

5. Optimize the ICU environment and make it peaceful and conducive to patient pain management. Play soft music the patient and family enjoy and offer guided imagery.

---

discharge and 43% having it 24 months after discharge. ICU diaries are also an emerging tool used in PICS prevention along with nutrition and ICU follow-up.[34,35] The nurse and care team keep intensive care diaries to record daily events to help orient the patient following discharge and have been shown to reduce anxiety, depression, and PTSD for patients and families.[35]

Follow-up care is essential for post-critical care patients to address needs and reduce PICS and help with chronic pain management. Studies show significant improvement in mental health, including PTSD and depression symptoms, with discharge follow-up (95% CI). Continuing education, evidence-based resources, including ICU diaries, support groups, and social service follow-ups help reduce the risk of PICS and other mental health conditions.[35]

SUMMARY

Patients in critical care may experience long-term physical, mental, and psychological effects. Unmanaged pain adds to the trauma. Multi-modal interventions of pharmacologic and nonpharmacologic complementary approaches help prevent long-term effects on the patient as well as improve the satisfaction of the family. Guided imagery and other complementary alternative methods, such as acupuncture, music and sound therapy, cold therapy, massage, and physical and occupational therapy, improve patient outcomes in intensive care.[1,2] Including the family and providing the patient and family with family-centered care, post-intensive care follow-up, and discharge resources can also reduce PICS, anxiety, depression, and PTSD.[35] As studies continue complementary alternative methods, critical care nurses aim to improve patient outcomes including reducing pain and anxiety in ICU patients.

CLINICS CARE POINTS

- Numerous assessment tools are available for critical nurses to assess the levels of pain, anxiety, and delirium in ICU patients.

- Using complementary approaches to address anxiety and pain in ICU-ventilated patients reduces hospital stays and poses fewer side effects than pain medication.

- Sedation and pain medication can be reduced with complementary therapies that can be implemented by nurses and the interdisciplinary ICU team.

DISCLOSURE

All authors report no commercial or financial conflicts of interest. There was no funding from any source for this publication.

REFERENCES

1. Nordness MF, Hayhurst CJ, Pandharipande P. Current Perspectives on the assessment and management of pain in the intensive care Unit. J Pain Res 2021;14:1733–44.
2. Zhang Y, Yang G, Wei J, et al. Prospective comparison of acupuncture with sham acupuncture to determine impact on sedation and analgesia in mechanically ventilated critically ill patients (PASSION study): Protocol for a randomized controlled trial. British Medical Journal Open 2022;12:e059741.
3. Jarvis C. Physical Examination & Health Assessment. 8th edition. Philadelphia, PA: W. B. Saunders; 2019.
4. Devlin JW, Skrobik Y, Gélinas C, et al. Clinical practice guidelines for the prevention and management of pain, agitation/sedation, delirium, immobility, and sleep disruption in adult patients in the ICU. Crit Care Med 2018;46(9):e825–73.
5. Gomarverdi S, Sedighie L, Seifrabiei MA, et al. Comparison of two pain scales: behavioral pain scale and critical-care pain Observation tool during Invasive and Noninvasive procedures in intensive care unit-admitted patients. Iran J Nurs Midwifery Res 2019;24(2):151–5.
6. Wilson DR, Pappas J, Taylor R. Hypnosis and pain. American Nurse Today; 2024.
7. Sandvik RK, Olsen BF, Lars-Jørgen R, et al. Pain relief from nonpharmacological interventions in the intensive care unit: a scoping review. J Clin Nurs 2020; 29(9–10):1488–98.
8. Krau SD. The Multiple Uses of guided imagery. Nurs Clin 2020;55(4):467–74. https://doi.org/10.1016/j.cnur.2020.06.013.
9. Cui N, Yan X, Zhang Y, et al. Nonpharmacological interventions for minimizing physical restraints Use in intensive care Units: an Umbrella review. Front Med 2022;9. https://doi.org/10.3389/fmed.2022.806945.
10. Parizad N, Gol R, Faraji N, et al. Effect of guided imagery on anxiety, muscle pain, and vital signs in patients with COVID-19. Compl Ther Clin Pract 2021; 43(101335). https://doi.org/10.1016/j.ctcp.2021.101335.
11. Hadjibalassi M, Lambrinou E, Papastavrou E, et al. The effect of guided imagery on physiological and psychological outcomes of adult ICU patients: a systematic literature review and methodological implications. Aust Crit Care 2018;31(2):73–86.
12. Thompson T, Terhune DB, Oram C, et al. The effectiveness of hypnosis for pain relief: a systematic review and meta-analysis of 85 controlled experimental trials. Neuroscience Biobehav Rev 2019;298–310.
13. World Health Organization. WHO Benchmarks for the practice of acupuncture. Available at: 2021 https://www.who.int/publications/i/item/978-92-4-001688-0. [Accessed 3 January 2024].
14. Chen T, Zhang WW, Chu YX, et al. Acupuncture for pain management: Molecular Mechanisms of action. Am J Chin Med 2020;48(4):793–811.
15. Witt CM, Pach D, Reinhold T, et al. Treatment of the adverse effects from acupuncture and their economic impact: a prospective study in 73,406 patients with low back or neck pain. Eur J Pain 2011;15:193–7.
16. Ben-Arie E, Lottering BJ, Chen FP, et al. Is acupuncture safe in the ICU? A systematic review and meta-analysis. Front Med 2023;10:1190635.

17. Dallı OE, Yıldırım Y, Aykar FS, et al. The effect of music on delirium, pain, sedation and anxiety in patients receiving mechanical ventilation in the intensive care unit. Intensive Crit Care Nurs 2023;75(103348). https://doi.org/10.1016/j.iccn.2022.103348.

18. Thenmozhi P, Indumathy S. Nature based sound therapy on pain and anxiety during extubation of mechanical ventilation. J Stage 2019;12:16–23.

19. Mohammadi N, Pooria A, Yarahmadi S, et al. Effects of cold application on chest tube removal pain in heart surgery patients. Tanaffos 2018;17(1):29–36.

20. Escalon MX, Lichtenstein AH, Posner E, et al. The effects of early mobilization on patients requiring Extended mechanical ventilation across Multiple ICUs. Critical Care Exploration 2020;2(6):e0119.

21. Wang YT, Lang J, Haines KJ, et al. Physical rehabilitation in the ICU: a systematic review and meta-analysis. Crit Care Med 2022;50(3):375–88.

22. Jagan S, Park T, Papathanassoglou E. Effects of massage on outcomes of adult intensive care unit patients: a systematic review. Nurs Crit Care 2019;24(6):414–29.

23. Vorona S, Sabatini U, Al-Maqbali S, et al. Inspiratory muscle rehabilitation in critically ill adults: a systematic review and meta-analysis. Annals of the American Thoracic Society 2018;15:735–44.

24. Harorani M, Garshasbi M, Sediqi M, et al. The effect of Shiatsu massage on agitation in mechanically ventilated patients: a randomized controlled trial. Heart Lung 2021;50(6):893–7.

25. Parhusip HL, Astrid M, Susilo WH. The effect of foot massage relaxation techniques to reduce pain level in patients with ventilator in ICU Cengkareng hospital in 2022. Asian Journal of Social and Humanities 2023;1(11). https://doi.org/10.59888/ajosh.v1i11.85.

26. Harlan EA, Miller J, Costa DK, et al. Emotional experiences and coping strategies of family members of critically ill patients. Chest 2020;158(4):1464–72.

27. Huang H, Dong H, Guan X, et al. The facilitated sensemaking model as a framework for nursing intervention on family members of mechanically ventilated patients in the intensive care unit. Worldviews Evidence-Based Nurs 2022;19(6):467–76.

28. Pinheiro I, Kohlsdorf M, Pérez-Nebra AR. Analysis of stress and coping in relatives of patients admitted to the ICU. Paideia 2022;32. https://doi.org/10.1590/1982-4327e3204.

29. Xyrichis A, Fletcher S, Philippou J, et al. Interventions to promote family member involvement in adult critical care settings: a systematic review. British Medical Journal Open 2021;11(4). https://doi.org/10.1136/bmjopen-2020-042556.

30. Cyran-Grzebyk B, Perenc L, Wyszyńska J, et al. The influence of family crisis coping strategies on family quality of life in the assessment of patients with idiopathic scoliosis. Int J Environ Res Publ Health 2023;20:1177.

31. Padilla-Fortunatti C, Munro C, Gattamorta K. Psychological distress, social support, and family satisfaction among family members of non-COVID-19 critical care patients: a cross-sectional study. Journal of Nursing Scholarship, Supplemental Special Issue: Health Policy Implications: Lessons Learned from Covid-19 2023;55(1):33–44.

32. Haave RO, Bakke HH, Schröder A. Family satisfaction in the intensive care unit, a cross-sectional study from Norway. BMC Emerg Med 2021;21(20). https://doi.org/10.1186/s12873-021-00412-8.

33. Schwartz AC, Dunn SE, Simon HFM, et al. Making family-centered care for adults in the ICU a reality. Front Psychiatr 2022;13:837708.

34. Vlake JH, van Genderen ME, Schut A, et al. Patients suffering from psychological impairments following critical illness are in need of information. J intensive care 2020;8(6). https://doi.org/10.1186/s40560-019-0422-0.
35. Inoue S, Hatakeyama J, Kondo Y, et al. Post-intensive care syndrome: its pathophysiology, prevention, and future directions. Acute Med Surg 2019;6: 233–46.

Managing Chronic Pain in Ventilated Critical Care Patients

Heather Moran, MSN, RN, CRRN, CMSRN, CNE,
Kristen Butler, DNP, MSN, RN*

KEYWORDS

- Chronic pain • Mechanically ventilated • Pain management • Pain
- Multimodal approaches • Pain assessment • ICU patients • Nurse

KEY POINTS

- A systematic, frequent pain assessment method incorporating self-report, behavioral evaluation, and family input should be used for mechanically ventilated patients.
- An appropriate, evidence-based pain assessment tool that assists in individualized pain assessments and management should be chosen.
- Prompt recognition and treatment of pain in the intensive care unit (ICU), along with rehabilitative strategies, can prevent chronic pain in ICU survivors.
- Evidence-based pain management protocols in the ICU should be established, emphasizing analgesia before sedation and aligning with the Society of Critical Care Medicine guidelines to improve patient outcomes.
- It is imperative to use multimodal strategies, including pharmacologic and nonpharmacologic interventions, to enhance pain relief and minimize pain-related complications in critically ill patients.

BACKGROUND/CONSIDERATIONS

Annually, there are more than 5 million intensive care unit (ICU) admissions in the United States, with an average length of stay of 3.8 days.[1] Consequently, most of these patients will experience moderate-to-severe pain during hospitalization and beyond discharge. ICU survivors are increasingly expressing that pain is one of their most disquieting memories of their hospitalization.[2] As Sandvik and colleagues reported[3] that approximately 50% of mechanically ventilated ICU patients experienced pain at rest and 81% experienced pain during a procedure. Pain, previously referred to as the "fifth vital sign" by the Joint Commission on Accreditation of Healthcare Organizations, is the biggest concern for patients.[4] The International Association for the

Austin Peay State University, 601 College Street, Clarksville, TN 37044, USA
* Corresponding author.
E-mail address: butlerk@apsu.edu

Crit Care Nurs Clin N Am 36 (2024) 553–566
https://doi.org/10.1016/j.cnc.2024.05.001   ccnursing.theclinics.com

Study of Pain defined pain as, "an unpleasant sensory and emotional experience associated with, or resembling that associated with, actual or potential tissue damage."[5] Additionally, an acute stress response is associated with pain, including psychological distress and changes to an individual's neurovegetative activity and neuroendocrine secretion, resulting in a variety of manifestations.[6]

The impact of pain during and following critical illness is profound, as it has been associated with post-traumatic stress disorder (PTSD), chronic pain, and poor quality of life.[7] Approximately 14% to 77% of ICU patients experience chronic pain following discharge.[7] Discomfort, defined as "negative emotional and/or physical state subject to variation in magnitude in response to internal or environmental conditions," often accompanies the pain experienced by patients.[8] Survivors of critical illness report long-term issues with physical, mental, and cognitive impairments known as post-intensive care syndrome (PICS).[7] Symptoms of PICS include chronic pain, weakness, fatigue, sleep deprivation, anxiety, depression, PTSD, and decline in memory, thinking, reasoning, problem-solving, and attentiveness.[9]

There is limited research on chronic pain during and after admission to the ICU. This article aims to explore the assessment and management of pain in mechanically ventilated critically ill patients, thus addressing persistent or chronic pain in ICU survivors. Current guidelines for pain management of critically ill patients do not differentiate treatment of acute versus chronic pain. However, with any type of pain, thorough, routine pain assessments and treatment protocols are critical in the treatment and management of pain in ventilated individuals.

ETIOLOGY OF PAIN IN INTENSIVE CARE UNIT PATIENTS

Critically ill patients frequently experience respiratory failure, resulting in the need for mechanical ventilation.[10] Patients receiving care in the ICU commonly experience pain due to numerous intrinsic and extrinsic factors.[8] Mechanical ventilation and other ICU-related invasive and noninvasive procedures are frequent sources of acute pain and discomfort. Critically ill patients experience inflammatory and ischemic pain related to their underlying and chronic conditions. Additionally, there are elements of neuropathic pain related to the presence of disease and secondary to procedures, surgeries, and trauma.[1] It has been hypothesized that ineffective assessment and management of acute pain is linked to the development of chronic pain.[7]

ETIOLOGY OF CHRONIC PAIN IN INTENSIVE CARE UNIT PATIENTS

Chronic pain is defined as pain that lasts beyond the usual or expected tissue healing time or pain lasting for 3 or more months without other causes or criteria.[11] When addressing chronic pain in critically ill patients, it is imperative to consider existing illness and disease prior to ICU admission. Approximately 21% of adults in the United States experience chronic pain, and approximately 7% experience high-impact chronic pain.[7] According to Kemp and colleagues,[7] chronic pain is most prevalent in ICU survivors (44.3%) compared to individuals not admitted to the ICU (25.7%). Painful preadmission comorbidities are correlated with the development of new-onset chronic pain following critical illness.[7] The incidence of new-onset chronic pain following ICU admission ranges between 22% and 33%.[7] One study exploring the most frequently reported sites of pain following ICU discharge found a 22% incidence of chronic shoulder pain.[7] Other body sites noted in the study to have a high incidence of post-ICU discharge pain include the spine, lower and upper limbs, abdomen, and pelvis.[7] Sepsis has also been linked to the development of chronic pain, suggesting that sustained inflammatory response is associated with neurologic damage.[7] In a systematic review conducted by Mäkinen and colleagues,[11] it was found that there was a high incidence of persistent pain (77%) 3 months after care in the ICU, with some individuals reporting pain 2 years after their hospitalization (36%). The review also revealed ICU-related patient risk factors for persistent pain, including organ failure, sepsis, pre-existing pain, and longer duration of mechanical ventilation or hospitalization.[11] Other risk factors associated with the development of chronic pain after ICU admission include age, ICU length of stay, and the presence and duration of mechanical ventilation.[9]

BARRIERS

The pain experience for an individual is complex. In the critical care setting, pain is frequently amplified by psychological distress, loss of sense of control, dependency on others, and limited or complete inability to communicate.[1] Factors that influence pain in critically ill adults include[12]

- Psychological factors such as anxiety and depression
- Demographic factors such as age, sex, ethnicity, comorbidities, and surgical history
- Type of procedure and intensity of related pain
- Surgical or medical diagnoses

Patients in critical care units are more likely to encounter barriers in expressing or verbalizing pain, discomfort, and suffering.[3] Owing to the presence of induced unconscious states, mechanical ventilation, brain injury, or intellectual deficits, the utilization of a self-reported pain scale is not conducive. This, however, does not exclude this population of patients from experiencing pain or necessitating pain relief. As a result, pain management in critically ill patients is difficult and can result in misuse of both sedatives and analgesics.[3]

Infrequent documentation of pain assessments by both nurses and providers and not using valid and reliable tools in critical care settings increase the likelihood of undetected patient pain and undertreatment.[13] The lack of knowledge and understanding of pain assessment tools also contributes to poor pain management. While the use of assessment tools and evidence-based guidelines to manage pain is recommended, it is noted that there is a decrease in adherence by health care providers to frequently and thoroughly assess pain among patients who cannot self-report pain.[2]

Sedation and analgesia have been the gold standard for the treatment of pain and discomfort in the ICU for many years. Analgesia has been used to manage pain, whereas sedation is often used to relieve stress, agitation, and anxiety in critically ill individuals.[5] Analgesia and sedation have been administered to assist with pain alleviation, optimize invasive procedure outcomes, decrease oxygen consumption, and improve synchronization with mechanical ventilation. However, oversedation and undersedation have been associated with prolonged hospitalizations and increased mortality rates.[13] New guidelines now focus on pain control with minimal use of sedation, resulting in improved patient outcomes.[5]

IMPACT

Studies report a global concern with the undertreatment of patient pain across all health care settings.[14] Ineffective pain management is associated with physical, psychological, and spiritual deficits.[14] Inadequate pain control is associated with delayed healing and the development of complications and contributes to the development of anxiety and sleep disorders.[14] Additionally, increased ICU length of stay, prolonged mechanical ventilation, PTSD, pulmonary complications, and patient–ventilator asynchrony can occur with uncontrolled pain, which can worsen the medical conditions and outcomes of patients.[1,6] Physiologic responses to pain can lead to potentially life-threatening complications such as unstable hemodynamic status, hyperglycemia, altered function of the immune system, and an increased release of the hormones catecholamine, cortisol, and antidiuretic hormone. Untreated or undertreated pain has been associated with an increase in morbidity and mortality.[2]

ROLE OF NURSE

Nurses play an essential role in the assessment and management of patient pain. However, studies report barriers such as knowledge and attitude concerning pain interfere with effective patient pain management.[14] In a cross-sectional study, Hamdan and colleagues noted the following barriers reported by nurses in the management of patient pain.[14]

- Nursing workload
- Patient instability
- Patient's inability to communicate
- Sedation restricting nurses' assessment of pain
- Lack of available pain assessment tools
- Lack of education/familiarity with pain assessment tools
- Inadequate prescribed analgesia
- Poor communication and documentation of pain and analgesia
- Poor prioritization of pain assessment
- Lack of ICU protocols and guidelines for the assessment of pain

Nurses' perceptions, knowledge, and beliefs also affect pain assessment practices and management. Nurses are continuously affected by their work culture, organizational structure, biases, ideas, and critical reflection.[13] Continuing education and professional development on evidence-based pain assessments and techniques should be integrated to increase knowledge transfer into nursing practice.[13] The American Society for Pain Management Nursing recommends nurses should encourage self-reporting of pain, be familiar with procedures that may cause pain or discomfort, monitor alterations in physiologic and behavioral factors of the patient, and follow protocols that establish the use of analgesics before sedation.[13] Appropriate assessment and management of pain in critically ill patients are linked to better patient outcomes, including early extubation and decreased delirium, ICU length of stay, use of sedation, and mortality rates.[1]

GOALS AND GUIDELINES OF PAIN MANAGEMENT

Pain management, including analgesia and sedation practices, for ICU patients is complex. Current practice standards in critical care environments support multimodal treatment plans.[4] Administering analgesia and sedation to mechanically ventilated patients supports patient comfort and safety; however, research reports that deep sedation is linked to prolonged mechanical ventilation, prolonged ICU and hospital stays, and increased mortality.[10] According to the Society of Critical Care Medicine (SCCM) Clinical Practice Guidelines for the Management of Pain, Agitation/Sedation, Delirium, Immobility, and Sleep Disruption in Adult Patients in the ICU (PADIS) published in 2018, the treatment of pain should be prioritized prior to administering sedation.[10,15] The 2018 PADIS guidelines recommend the administration of sedation once adequate analgesia is achieved. Not all mechanically ventilated patients require sedation; however, sedatives offer additional support to promote comfort, safety, and patient–ventilator synchrony.[10]

Current guidelines for pain management in the ICU emphasize the importance of a multimodal regimen. The 2018 PADIS guidelines and the ICU liberation bundle published by the SCCM provide relevant, evidenced-based clinical resources and recommendations to address pain, agitation/sedation, delirium, immobility, and sleep disruption.[12,15] The ICU liberation bundle overview can be found and downloaded from https://sccmmedia.sccm.org/video/OnlineCourse/ICU-Liberation-A-F-Bundle-Overview/story.html. According to the SCCM, the components of the guidelines are interrelated; therefore, each should not be independently implemented.[12,15] The SCCMs ICU liberation bundle supports a holistic approach to implementing the PADIS guidelines.[15] One element of the ICU liberation bundle emphasizes assessment, prevention, and intervention for pain management.[15] Adequate pain management strategies begin with assessment and include communication and use of validated pain assessment tools such as, but not limited to, the numeric rating scale (NRS), behavioral pain scale (BPS), and the critical care pain observation tool (CPOT).[15]

ASSESSMENT OF PAIN IN INTENSIVE CARE UNIT PATIENTS

Adequate assessment of pain in ICU patients is essential to proper management, resulting in overall better short- and long-term outcomes. Assessments are integral to gaining valuable insight and knowledge to guide complex decision-making, especially in the ICU.[13] Pain assessments can be difficult due to the subjectivity of pain, whether acute or chronic, and usually only measured when the individual reports it. However, as mentioned previously, the critically ill who may be sedated and ventilated cannot report or describe their pain.[16]

To adequately assess pain in sedated and ventilated patients, nurses must take a multifaceted approach, including analysis of physiologic responses, physical behaviors, pain scores, family perspectives, and patient baselines. Assessments must also include sound clinical judgment to differentiate between patient situations that require analgesia versus sedation.[13] Furthermore, assessment and understanding of a patient's chronic pain is necessary to manage those experiences along with episodes of acute pain that may be elicited during hospitalization. Thorough questions regarding ongoing, chronic pain should be included in health history evaluations to gain a better understanding of the patient's baseline experiences, perceptions, and management of pain. Families and caregivers may need to be included in these initial assessments if the patient is sedated, ventilated, and/or unable to respond. It is also recommended that the family be included in all subsequent pain assessments as warranted and necessary.[13]

Assessments of pain should be completed frequently, usually at least every 2 hours, in critical care areas, with reassessments occurring within 1 hour after any intervention has been made.[15] The ICU liberation bundle outlines a stepwise approach to pain assessment and suggests conducting assessments in the following order.

1. Attempt to obtain self-report pain
2. Assess for behavioral changes
3. Ask family or caregivers to assist in identifying pain behaviors
4. Assume pain is present

It is recommended to use an assessment-driven, protocol-based, stepwise, multifaceted approach for pain, analgesia, and sedation management.[13]

MANIFESTATIONS OF PAIN

Pain can manifest in individuals in various ways. Besides the verbalization of pain, behavioral changes can also indicate pain and discomfort. Mechanically ventilated patients are typically sedated, unconscious, and unable to self-report pain experiences. Therefore, it is essential to understand and recognize common behavioral changes that can be observed and signify pain.[16] Observing changes in facial expressions is one of the most common methods used to assess ventilated patients. During painful experiences and procedures, an increase in facial movements can occur, including closed eyes, brows furrowed or lowered, raised cheeks, parted lips, tightened eyelids, and grimacing.[15,16] Additionally, an increase in body movements (restlessness), muscle rigidity, compliance with mechanical ventilation, and sounds can be other behavior indicators of pain and its intensity.[15,16]

PAIN ASSESSMENT TOOLS/SCALES

Numerous pain assessment tools have been developed and used across all health care settings. Frequent, routine pain assessments using valid and reliable scales/tools assist health care providers in understanding a patient's overall status, guide decisions about pain management, and enhance the possibility of adequate pain control and avoidance of breakthrough pain.[13] It is essential to utilize the most appropriate assessment tool for each individual patient, considering their cognitive abilities, behaviors, visual, verbal, and auditory limitations, and sedation and ventilation status.[16] The most commonly valid and reliable pain assessment tools, along with some newer upcoming tools for this patient population, are discussed in the following sections.

Self-Reporting: Numerical, Visual, and PQRSTUV

The gold standard pain assessment tool is the subjective self-reporting tool. The most common self-reporting tool used is the NRS. The NRS is a self-reporting pain method that allows the individual to rate their pain on a scale, typically 0 to 10, with 0 representing no pain and 10 representing a significant amount of pain or severe pain.[1] Patients who are sedated or nonverbal cannot self-report pain on the NRS. The numeric pain rating scale-visual component (NRS-V) is an adapted version of the NRS, where a visualization of the scale is shown. The visual component allows the scale to be shown in large font with the numbers 0 to 10 and explanations, such as "no pain" and "severe pain" or extreme pain, next to the associated number.[1] Intubated patients who are not sedated or nonverbal patients can use the NRS-V by pointing to their corresponding pain level with the visualization of the NRS shown to them.[1] The NRS and NRS-V can be found and downloaded from https://www.sccm.org/sccm/media/PDFs/Pain-Numeric-Rating-Scale-Enlarged.pdf.[15]

In addition to the patients self-reporting their pain and placing a numerical value on it, nurses should also encourage using the mnemonic PQRSTUV to help characterize the pain. PQRSTUV stands for: P, pain factors and causes; Q, pain quality or sensation; R, pain region or location; S, pain severity or intensity; T, pain duration, frequency, or temporality; U, understand previous pain experiences and problems; and V, patient values, beliefs, and preferences of pain and treatment.[1] This mnemonic is extremely helpful in identifying causes, location, timeframes, and pain-relieving values, preferences, and strategies of the patient. It is highly encouraged and expected for health care providers, especially nurses, to conduct a thorough pain assessment upon arrival and admission to the ICU.[1]

While self-reporting is ideal and the gold standard, it does not come without its limitations. Oral and visual self-reporting scales have practical limitations. They should not be used on patients with delirium, visual or hearing impairment, and anyone who cannot follow commands or instructions.[1] Furthermore, as mentioned, sedated, mechanically ventilated, and some critically ill patients cannot verbalize their pain, and other available evidence-based scales should be used.

Behavioral/Objective Pain Scales

Objective or behavioral observational scales are the second choice after self-reporting. Behavioral assessment tools can be used for critically ill patients unable to report pain due to a variety of reasons, such as sedation, ventilation, and delirium, among other issues.[1] These types of tools use observations of patient behaviors, physiologic parameters, especially changes in vital signs, and possibly other body signs as objective measures for pain, as it is understood that behavioral responses are directly proportional to pain intensity scores.[16]

These assessment instruments can be unidimensional or multidimensional. A single dimension (eg, behavioral responses) is used in a unidimensional scale, incorporating one (only facial expressions) or multiple (facial expressions, sounds, and body movements) domains in the evaluation of the patient.[16] On the other hand, multidimensional tools incorporate at least two pain dimensions, such as behaviors and physiologic responses, and usually have several domains within each category. Additionally, multidimensional scales must use the clinical judgment of nurses and other health care providers.[16] While these behavior tools are not directly interchangeable with self-reported pain, they have been validated in numerous critically ill patient populations.[1] The CPOT and BPS are available in numerous different languages and have shown robust psychometric performance, becoming the most translated, validated, and reliable behavioral pain assessment tools.[6,13,17]

Vital signs

For many decades, it has been thought vital sign variations, including heart rate, blood pressure, and respirations, were sufficient for predicting and assessing pain in critically ill patients who could not verbalize their pain or discomfort. While these parameters are frequently still used in critical care areas, vital signs are not an adequate pain assessment tool, as nonpainful experiences, physiologic stressors, and underlying disease pathology can contribute to fluctuations in these monitoring parameters.[1] There can be a wide range of physiologic changes and variations in critically ill patients, such as tachycardia, tachypnea, and hypotension or hypertension that are completely unrelated to painful stimuli. Still, health care providers often inappropriately attribute these changes to pain.[1,13] Therefore, vital signs should not be used solely for pain assessments; however, they can serve as cues for nurses and other health care providers to conduct further pain assessments.[1,6,12]

Critical care pain observation tool

The CPOT is one of the most used behavioral pain assessment scales for patients who are unable to self-report. Numerous studies on many patient populations supported inter-rater reliability, internal consistency, sensitivity, specificity, feasibility, and validity, confirming its effectiveness in the ICU with sedated and ventilated, and nonintubated patients.[13,16] Four behaviors are assessed when using the CPOT: facial expressions, movements, muscle tension, and ventilator compliance. Each behavioral domain is scored 0 to 2 based on observations with a total score of 0 (no pain) to 8 (severe or most pain) and a score greater than 2 indicating an unacceptable level of pain.[1,16] A previous study initiating a pain measurement routine using the CPOT positively influenced pain assessments and management. Pain assessments and documentation of pain-indicative behaviors were reported, resulting in a decreased use of analgesics, propofol, and morphine boluses.[16] The CPOT pain assessment tool can be found at https://www.mdcalc.com/calc/2144/critical-care-pain-observation-tool-cpot.[15]

Behavioral pain scale

Another commonly used behavior pain assessment scale is the BPS. The BPS has 3 behavioral domains: facial expressions, upper limb movement, and mechanical ventilation compliance.[1,16] Using the BPS is supported by the tool's internal consistency, inter-rater reliability, sensitivity, specificity, and validity.[16] Each behavior domain is scored 1 to 4 based on observations with a total score of 3 (no pain) to 12 (severe or most pain) and a score greater than or equal to 6 indicating pain that should be addressed and treated.[1,16] Implementing the BPS in ICUs has increased pain assessment frequency and improved pain management and patient outcomes.[16] The BPS pain assessment tool for intubated patients can be found at https://www.mdcalc.com/calc/3622/behavioral-pain-scale-bps-pain-assessment-intubated-patients.[15]

Pupillometry. A newer method of pain assessment is using pupillometry. Pupillometry can assist in assessing pupil reaction to medications and other noxious stimuli.[13] It can be used in the titration of analgesics and anesthesia as it can detect the effects of opioids and other medications. In one study, an increase in pupil size by 16% was noted in sedated and ventilated patients during noxious procedures.[13] In another study conducted in the ICU, the presence of pain was detected with a pupil size variation of greater than 19% with a specificity of 77% and sensitivity of 100%.[13] However, further research is needed to identify the reliability and validity in more ICU settings and patient populations.[13]

MANAGEMENT OF PAIN

Prevention of patient pain involves early recognition of the potential of pain with standard ICU procedures such as patient positioning, removal of drains (ie, chest tubes, wound drains), wound care, and indwelling line insertion (ie, intravenous catheters, arterial lines, chest tubes, Foley catheters). Interventions for pain management include both nonpharmacologic and pharmacologic interventions. Nonpharmacologic interventions include family support, pet therapy, music therapy, massage and touch practices, education/teaching, relaxation, and distraction techniques.[15] Nonpharmacologic approaches have gained significant traction in the management of physical, sensory, emotional, affective, and cognitive effects of pain.[1] Pharmacologic strategies have been the foundation of pain management in critically ill patients in the ICU; however, side effects such as respiratory depression, sedation, opioid tolerance, ileus, withdrawal, and delirium must be considered.[15]

PHARMACOLOGIC INTERVENTIONS
Analgesia

Opioids continue to be the drug of choice for pain management in critically ill patients in the ICU setting and are prioritized before initiating sedation therapy.[15] Intravenously administered morphine, hydromorphone, fentanyl, and remifentanil are among the most commonly prescribed opioid analgesics used for pain control in mechanically ventilated ICU patients.[10] Nonopioid analgesics such as acetaminophen, ibuprofen, nefopam, lidocaine, nonsteroidal anti-inflammatory drugs, and neuropathic agents may be used as adjuvant therapy to enhance reduction of pain and minimize the use of opioids.[15] According to the SCCM, opioids are the first choice for the management of non-neuropathic pain.[1,15] However, pain management strategies should correspond with pain assessment tools, thus using titration protocols based on pain scores.[1] The utilization of evidence-based, standardized assessment tools and pain management protocols has been associated with lower doses of opioids and effective pharmacologic pain relief.[1] The use of analgesia and sedation for the treatment of pain must be carefully approached. The excessive use of analgesia and sedation and untreated patient pain are associated with an increased risk for ICU delirium. The long-term impact of ICU delirium contributes to PICS.[1]

Sedation

A common misconception of sedated ICU patients is that they do not have an awareness of pain; however, many studies discredit this myth with patient reports of vivid memories of their ICU experiences.[1] According to the guidelines, sedation is only to be administered once analgesia has been adequately achieved.[10] Sedation for mechanically ventilated patients is not always necessary with adequate pain control; however, sedation can enhance patient comfort, safety, and patient–ventilator synchrony.[10] The administration of sedation to mechanically ventilated ICU patients should follow algorithms that use validated agitation and pain scales and incorporate daily sedation interruptions or nonsedation practices.[10] Commonly prescribed sedative medications for ICU patients include benzodiazepines, propofol, and dexmedetomidine. Careful titration of sedative medications should be implemented to avoid oversedation. Daily sedation interruption practices have been associated with early extubation, decreased ICU length of stay, decreased complications, and improved overall patient outcomes.[10]

NONPHARMACOLOGIC INTERVENTIONS

Although the use of pharmacologic approaches for the management of pain in the ICU is effective, there are significant short- and long-term adverse effects. The use of nonpharmacologic approaches for pain management has become more mainstream in recent years and has been integrated into the 2018 PADIS guidelines.[15] Nonpharmacologic approaches for the management of pain have minimal adverse effects and are considered safer and more convenient than the use of pharmacologic therapies.[18] In the ICU, acute pain is a primary focus of concern. Nonetheless, unrelieved acute pain is a significant risk factor for the development of chronic pain and PICS, and it contributes to poor patient outcomes and is a source of distress for patients.[19] The 2018 PADIS guidelines and ICU liberation bundle promote the following nonpharmacologic interventions for pain management.[15]

- Massage therapy
- Music and sound therapy
- Cold therapy
- Relaxation techniques

Nonpharmacologic approaches can be used independently and complementarily and have other advantages, such as reduced hospital costs, increased patient satisfaction, and decreased likelihood of drug dependence.[18]

Massage Therapy

Studies support the use of massage to enhance pain management in ICU patients.[20] In a randomized-controlled trial (RCT) of surgical cardiac ICU patients, hand massage interventions yielded significantly lower pain intensity scores, pain unpleasantness scores, and reduced anxiety levels.[20] In a parallel, single-bind RCT of trauma ICU patients, intervention groups who received a 6 day Swedish foot massage from nurses and family members had statistically significant lower pain mean scores compared to the control group.[21] According to the ICU Liberation Bundle,[15] massage therapy can be performed on the hands, feet, and back. Massages can be performed by massage therapists, trained nursing staff, and/or family members (with guidance from staff).[1] Massages consist of approximately 20 minutes of light pressure at least twice daily. To maximize the benefits of massage, it is recommended to combine with decreasing sensory stimuli such as reducing light (ie, eye mask, dim lights) and sounds (ie, earplugs, mute alarms, lower volumes).[1]

Music and Sound Therapy

The 2018 PADIS guidelines suggest integrating music therapy to assist in managing both procedural and nonprocedural pain in critically ill patients.[15] ICU settings are full of loud devices and alarms, often disturbing the rest and sleep of patients. Noisy environments also have an impact on patient pain, comfort, anxiety, and agitation levels.[22] Studies have demonstrated that nonpharmacologic interventions such as music and sound therapy have been effective in decreasing heart rate, blood pressure, anxiety, agitation, and pain in mechanically ventilated patients.[23] Further, music interventions have demonstrated effectiveness in managing the mental, physical, emotional, and social needs of patients.[24] Golino and colleagues explored the effects of live music therapy on adult mechanically ventilated ICU patients and noted improved pain and agitation scores.[23] Several strategies to decrease the effect of environmental noises on patient outcomes have been studied including the use of noise-canceling headphones and relaxing music therapy.[22] In a mixed method study of adult critically ill patients, Fallek and colleagues noted a decrease in pain and anxiety levels and a decrease in respiratory and pulse rates following music therapy sessions.[23] The evidence denotes that music therapy provides many benefits without the risk and may prevent ICU delirium.[23]

Cold Therapy

The 2018 PADIS guidelines support the use of cold therapy for procedural pain management in ICU patients.[15] Cold therapy interventions have effectively reduced procedural pain.[3] Cold ice packs placed 10 to 15 minutes prior to procedures were associated with lower pain scores.[1] Procedures such as chest tube removals, venipuncture, cardioversion, and breathing/coughing exercises were noted in several studies to have used cold therapy for preprocedural pain intervention.[19] Cold therapy, or cryotherapy, is a commonly used therapeutic application to treat both chronic and acute pain and is used for managing hemorrhage, swelling, and inflammation.[25] Cryotherapy involves the superficial, local, and nonlocal application of ice packs, baths, wraps, massage, and vapocoolant sprays.[25] The benefits of cold therapy include ease of use, inexpensive, and minimal adverse effects.[25]

Relaxation Techniques

Nonpharmacologic relaxation approaches such as guided imagery, breathing exercises, hypnosis, and biofeedback have been used in the management of pain in critically ill patients.[1] Relaxation-focused interventions promote a sense of calmness and stimulate responses that support a reduction in pain and stress.[26] Guided imagery is a practice that engages patients in a relaxed state where they mentally visualize peaceful and positive images.[27] In a systematic literature review, Hadjibalassi and colleagues noted several studies where implementing guided imagery practices in critically ill patients reduced the use of pharmacologic pain medication approaches.[27]

Additionally, several studies employing guided imagery in ICU patients reported decreased anxiety levels, systolic blood pressure, ICU length of stay, medical costs, and increased patient satisfaction.[27] In a quasi-experimental study of post-cardiac artery bypass graft patients in the ICU, deep breathing exercises were provided 5 minutes prior to and during the removal of chest tubes (to include the removal of dressings and sutures).[28] Perceived levels of pain in the intervention and control groups were collected and recorded at 5 minutes prior to removal and 5 and 15 minutes immediately after removal.[28] Pain levels recorded at 5 minutes prior to removal did not vary significantly between the control and intervention groups; however, the intervention group reported lower perceived pain levels at 5 and 15 minutes after removal compared to the control group.[28]

CHRONIC PAIN MANAGEMENT IN INTENSIVE CARE UNIT SURVIVORS

Management of chronic pain after ICU discharge (chronic post ICU pain [CPIP]) remains an important issue, as the incidence of post-ICU chronic pain ranges between 22% and 73%.[9] Chronic pain, often referred to as persistent pain, affects patients for months and years beyond ICU discharge.[7] Studies exploring pain intensity in ICU survivors found that greater than 50% of patients report moderate-to-severe levels of pain that are both disabling and restrict daily living activities.[7] CPIP was found to interfere with physical, psychological, and social well-being and interfere with daily activities such as employment, physical activity, relationships, attitude, behavior, and sleep.[9] CPIP is a major risk factor for chronic opioid use.[9] Chronic opioid use is defined as "daily or near-daily use of opioids for at least 90 days, often indefinitely."[9] The literature supports preventive measures to reduce the risk of CPIP, including effective management of acute pain in the ICU setting.[9] Additionally, Stamenkovic and colleagues[9] recommend a timely, comprehensive follow-up to evaluate for CPIP after ICU discharge to ensure appropriate pain management and implementation of physical and cognitive rehabilitative strategies.

RECOMMENDATIONS AND FUTURE DIRECTIONS

The decreased amount of research associated with chronic pain in ventilated patients increases the difficulty of having evidence-based practices that guide health care providers, especially nurses. Analysis of the pain assessment practices used for ventilated patients, specifically for chronic pain in critical care areas, and identification of all the barriers that hinder nurses and providers from properly assessing and managing pain in these patients is greatly needed. With further research, standardized, routine pain assessments can, and should, be established in ICU settings with treatment protocols and guidelines outlined based on repetitive assessments.[13,16] Frequent pain assessments using structured, validated, reliable, and feasible tools assist nurses in formulating individualized pain management plans, as it has been shown to improve consistency and patient outcomes.[1,13,16]

A multidisciplinary approach is necessary for adequate pain management. Pain assessments and management are indicated for all ICU health care professionals, specifically those individuals who directly care for the patients, such as providers, clinicians, nurses, and physical and occupational therapists.[16] Increased standardized education on the proper use of assessment tools and pain management guidelines is indicated for nurses and other health care providers to increase consistency and compliance, thus resulting in better patient outcomes. Furthermore, family member engagement and adequate interprofessional communication are also recommended.[13]

SUMMARY

The prevalence of pain in critically ill patients, particularly those undergoing mechanical ventilation, is a significant concern. Chronic pain during hospitalization and following ICU discharge is a complex issue, influenced by various factors, including pre-existing conditions and ICU-related interventions. Barriers to pain assessment persist, necessitating a multidimensional approach. Nurses play a pivotal role yet face challenges in assessing sedated patients. Adequate pain management is crucial for improved patient outcomes, emphasizing the importance of following evidence-based guidelines and utilizing appropriate assessment tools. The multifaceted nature of pain underscores the need for a comprehensive and individualized approach in critical care settings. Effective pain management in the ICU requires a holistic approach, combining opioids with nonopioid analgesics and nonpharmacologic strategies such as music and massage. The incidence of chronic pain post-ICU discharge emphasizes the need for preventive measures and a multidisciplinary approach. Standardized assessments and ongoing research are crucial for advancing evidence-based practices in ICU pain management.

CLINICS CARE POINTS

- Adopt a stepwise pain assessment approach, covering self-report, behavioral assessments and family input for intubated patients when conducting regular assessments at least every 2 hours, with postintervention reassessments conducted after 1 hour to guide pain management decisions.

- Select the most suitable pain assessment tool, considering patient characteristics, such as cognitive abilities and sedation status, utilizing validated and reliable tools such as NRS, BPS, or COPT.

- Advocate for the integration of evidence-based pain management protocols in the ICU, emphasizing prioritizing analgesia before sedation in alignment with the SCCM guidelines to enhance patient outcomes, including reduced ICU length of stay and mortality rates.

- Multimodal approaches, integrating opioids with nonopioid analgesics and nonpharmacologic interventions, are supported by evidence to optimize pain relief while mitigating opioid-associated risks in critically ill patients.

- Timely recognition and management of acute pain in the ICU are vital to prevent chronic pain in survivors, necessitating thorough post-ICU discharge follow-up for chronic pain evaluation and rehabilitative strategy implementation.

DISCLOSURE

All authors report no commercial or financial conflicts of interest. There was no funding from any source for this publication.

REFERENCES

1. Nordness MF, Hayhurst CJ, Pandharipande P. Current perspectives on the assessment and management of pain in the intensive care unit. J Pain Res 2021;14:1733–44.
2. Ayasrah SM. Pain among non-verbal critically ill mechanically ventilated patients: prevalence, correlates, and predictors. J Crit Care 2019;49:14–20.
3. Sandvik RK, Olsen BF, Rygh L, et al. Pain relief from nonpharmacological interventions in the intensive care unit: a scoping review. J Clin Nurs 2020;29:1488–98.

4. Wyler D, Esterlis M, Dennie BB, et al. Challenges of pain management in neurologically injured patients: systematic review protocol of analgesia and sedation strategies for early recovery from neurointensive care. Syst Rev 2018;7:104.

5. Ashkenazy S, Weissman C, Ganz FD. Perception of discomfort by mechanical ventilation patient in the intensive care unit: a qualitative study. Intensive Crit Care Nurs 2021;64(103016):103016.

6. Pota V, Coppolino F, Barbarisi A, et al. Pain in intensive care: a narrative review. Pain and Therapy 2022;11:359–67.

7. Kemp HI, Laycock H, Costello A, et al. Chronic pain in critical care survivors: a narrative review. Br J Anaesth 2019;123(2):372–84.

8. Luckhardt EM, Gunnels MS, Chlan LL. Assessing discomfort in critically ill patients: a narrative review of the literature. Crit Care Nurse 2022;42(4):47–54.

9. Stamenkovic DM, Laycock H, Karanikolas M, et al. Chronic pain and chronic opioid use after intensive care discharge – is it time to change practice? Front Pharmacol 2019;10:23.

10. Pearson SD, Patel BK. Evolving targets for sedation during mechanical ventilation. Curr Opin Crit Care 2020;26(1):47–52.

11. Mäkinen OJ, Bäcklund ME, Liisanantti J, et al. Persistent pain in intensive care survivors: a systemic review. Br J Anaesth 2020;125(2):149–58.

12. Devlin JW, Skrobik Y, Gelinas C, et al. Clinical practice guidelines for the prevention and management of pain, agitation/sedation, delirium, immobility, and sleep disruption in adult patients in the ICU. Crit Care Med 2018;46(9):825–73.

13. Kerbage SH, Garvey L, Lambert GW, et al. Pain assessment of the adult sedated and ventilated patients in the intensive care setting: a scoping review. Int J Nurs Stud 2021;122(104044):104004.

14. Hamdan KM, Shaheen AM, Abdalrahim MS. Barriers and enablers of intensive care unit nurses' assessment and management of patients' pain. Nurs Crit Care 2021;27:567–75.

15. Society of Critical Care Medicine. ICU liberation bundle (A-F). 2018. Available at: https://www.sccm.org/ICULiberation/ABCDEF-Bundles.

16. Azevedo-Santos IF, DeSanta JM. Pain measurement techniques: spotlight on mechanically ventilated patients. J Pain Res 2018;11:2969–80.

17. Chanques G, Gélinas C. Monitoring pain in the intensive care unit (ICU). Intensive Care Med 2022;48:1508–11.

18. Kia Z, Allahbakhshian M, Ilkhani M, et al. Nurses' use of non-pharmacological pain management methods in intensive care units: a descriptive cross-sectional study. Compl Ther Med 2021;58:102705.

19. Martorella G. Characteristics of nonpharmacological interventions for pain management in the ICU: a scoping review. Advanced Critical Care 2019;30(4):388–97.

20. Boitor M, Martorella G, Maheu C, et al. Effects of massage in reducing pain and anxiety of the cardiac surgery critically ill – a randomized controlled trial. Pain Med 2018;19:2556–69.

21. Momeni M, Arab M, Dehghan M, et al. The effect of foot massage on pain of the intensive care patients: a parallel randomized single-blind controlled trial. Evid base Compl Alternative Med 2020;3450853. https://doi.org/10.1155/2020/3450853.

22. Mateu-Capell M, Arnau A, Juvinya D, et al. Sound isolation and music on the comfort of mechanically ventilated critical patients. Nurs Crit Care 2018;24(5):290–8.

23. Golino AJ, Leone R, Gollenberg A, et al. Receptive music therapy for patients receiving mechanical ventilation in the intensive care unit. Am J Crit Care 2023; 32(2):109–15.
24. Fallek R, Corey K, Zamar A, et al. Soothing the heart with music: a feasibility study of a bedside music therapy intervention for critically ill patients in an urban hospital setting. Palliat Support Care 2019;18:47–54.
25. Garcia C, Karri J, Zacharias NA, et al. Use of cryotherapy for managing chronic pain: an evidenced-based narrative. Pain and Therapy 2021;10:81–100.
26. Papathanassoglou EDE, Hadjibalassi M, Panagiota M, et al. Effects of an integrative nursing intervention on pain in critically ill patients: a pilot clinical trial. Am J Crit Care 2018;27(3):172–85.
27. Hadjibalassi M, Lambrinou E, Papstavrou E, et al. The effect of guided imagery on physiological and psychological outcomes of adult ICU patients: a systematic literature review and methodological implications. Aust Crit Care 2018;31:73–86.
28. Jarrah MI, Hweidi IM, Al-Dolat SA, et al. The effect of slow deep breathing relaxation exercise on pain levels during and post chest removal after coronary artery bypass graft surgery. Int J Nurs Sci 2022;9:155–61.

Moral Distress and Pain Management
Implications for Critical Care Nurses

Preston H. Miller, PhD, RN, CCRN-CMC, PCCN, CFRN

KEYWORDS

- Moral distress • Ethics • Critical care • Nursing • Pain management • Well-being

KEY POINTS

- Moral distress is an unavoidable phenomenon that critical care nurses face in practice.
- If left unaddressed, or ineffectively addressed, moral distress can result in critical care nurses experiencing burnout, compassion fatigue, and leaving their role or the profession.
- Critical care nurses managing patient pain should be aware of the ethical and moral issues associated with pain management to develop and maintain resilience.
- Critical care nurse leaders and hospital administrators should incorporate strategies to identify, address, and mitigate moral distress among nurses associated with pain management and other contributing factors to moral distress.

INTRODUCTION

Pain management is a routine aspect of care for most patients in the critical care setting. The International Association for the Study of Pain defines pain as: "An unpleasant sensory and emotional experience associated with, or resembling that associated with, actual or potential tissue damage."[1] In 2019, the American Nurses Association[2] (ANA) published a position statement regarding the ethical responsibility of nurses to manage the pain and the suffering it causes. Within the position statement, several barriers to providing ethical pain management are noted. These barriers include moral disengagement, knowledge deficits, biases, environments not conducive to optimal practice, and economic limitations.[2] To address these barriers, the ANA recommends several strategies targeted at recognizing and acknowledging biases associated with pain management, developing moral courage and resiliency, pain management education, and the formation of collaboratives with providers to address substance-use disorder.[2] Critical care nurses may experience moral distress resulting from constraints encountered in practice that prevent them from managing pain in an ethically appropriate manner.

Department of Nursing, University of Alabama in Huntsville College of Nursing, 1410 Ben Graves Drive Northwest, Nursing Building 207B, Huntsville, AL 35805, USA
E-mail address: phm0002@uah.edu

Crit Care Nurs Clin N Am 36 (2024) 567–574
https://doi.org/10.1016/j.cnc.2024.04.011
0899-5885/24/© 2024 Elsevier Inc. All rights reserved.

ccnursing.theclinics.com

Moral distress as a phenomenon was first defined by Professor Andrew Jameton[3] in 1984 as, "when one knows the right thing to do, but institutional constraints make it nearly impossible to pursue the right course of action." Our understanding of moral distress has evolved since the inception of the phenomenon and several definitions exist within the literature. For the purposes of this article, moral distress is defined as occurring when nurses are constrained from taking ethically appropriate actions they perceive as correct or are forced to take ethically inappropriate actions which conflict with their professional obligations, resulting in feelings of complicity and wrongdoing.[4–7] The experience of moral distress can have an array of negative physical, psychological, and emotional effects[8,9] (**Table 1**) and may ultimately result in burnout, compassion fatigue, and nurses leaving their roles or the profession.[10–12] Nurses, especially those working in critical care settings, may experience moral distress at greater frequencies and intensities than nurses working in other settings[13] as well as other health care professionals.[14] To effectively advocate for patients and patient families, it is imperative for critical care nurses to be familiar with the ethical and moral challenges associated with pain management. The purpose of this clinical review article is to describe the current understanding of moral distress and pain management and identify practical implications for critical care nurses, critical care nurse leaders, and leaders of organizations.

PAIN IN THE CRITICAL CARE SETTING

Studies suggest that the incidence of pain in the critical care setting approaches 50% for both medical and surgical patients.[15] Patients may experience pain due to a variety of causes stemming from critical illness, invasive treatment(s), and procedures.[16] Critical care-related procedures such as arterial line insertion and chest tube and drain removal are viewed as most painful among critically ill patients, while mechanical ventilation, endotracheal tube suctioning, and repositioning have been noted to be uncomfortable

Table 1
Depicts the emotional, physical, and psychological symptoms of moral distress[8,9]

Category	Symptom
Emotional	• Anger • Anxiety • Frustration • Guilt • Irritability • Powerlessness • Sadness • Withdrawal
Physical	• Muscle aches • Headaches • Heart palpitations • Neck pain • Diarrhea • Vomiting
Psychological	• Depression • Emotional exhaustion • Loss of self-worth • Nightmares • Decreasing job satisfaction • Depersonalization of patients

among critically ill patients.[17] Pain in the critical care setting can be assessed via a variety of methods. These methods include both self-report and observed pain scales, such as the numeric rating scale and behavioral pain scale, and are considered quality, evidence-based tools by clinical practice recommendations.[18]

The Society of Critical Care Medicine's (SCCM) 2018 *Clinical Practice Guidelines for the Prevention and Management of Pain, Agitation/Sedation, Delirium, Immobility, and Sleep Disruption in Adult Patients in the ICU*[18] outlines a variety of recommendations pertinent to the management of pain exhibited by adult critical care patients. One key recommendation is that "the management of pain for adult intensive care unit (ICU) patients should be guided by routine pain assessment and pain should be treated before a sedative agent is considered."[18(pe837)] In summary, other recommendations are for health care professionals to accurately and effectively identify risk factors for pain, measuring pain using valid and reliable methods, providers to consider adjuvants to opioid therapy, the use of pharmacologic interventions to manage procedural pain, and the use of nonpharmacologic interventions to manage pain.[18] Additionally, the SCCMs 2022 *PANDEM Guidelines for Infants and Children*[19] outlines pain management recommendations for pediatric populations. Critical care nurses should familiarize themselves with the SCCM clinical practice guidelines relevant to pain management as a means to both educate and equip themselves with the information needed to serve as advocates for their patients when issues arise surrounding the management of patient pain.

MORAL DISTRESS IN THE CRITICAL CARE SETTING

In workforce studies conducted by Ulrich and colleagues,[20–24] moral distress has been noted as a primary issue affecting turnover, retention, and the well-being of critical care nurses. The most recent report was published in 2022 and detailed survey results from 2021 at the height of the COVID-19 pandemic. The percentage of participants who reported experiencing moral distress "very frequently" has consistently risen with each report; however, the percentage doubled from 11% to 22% in the 2022 report.[24] While moral distress has been heavily studied among bedside critical care nurses, recent studies suggest that critical care nurse leaders also experience the phenomenon.[25] Precipitating factors of moral distress in the critical care setting include issues regarding end-of-life care and decision-making,[26] lack of resources, unclear goals of care, and inconsistencies with treatment plans.[27] Issues surrounding pain management may also contribute to critical care nurses' experience of moral distress.[28]

MORAL DISTRESS AND PAIN MANAGEMENT

Literature surrounding the relationship of pain management and moral distress is limited. Of the studies identified for this review, moral distress was associated with managing the pain of patients at the end of life and patients with cancer. Additionally, pain caused by medication and/or treatment—*iatrogenic pain*—has also been identified as a source of moral distress among nurses.

Challenges associated with caring for patients at the end of life are a well-known and studied source of moral distress among nurses.[29] In regard to pain management, moral distress may be experienced by nurses when there is uncertainty regarding the effectiveness of pain management in relieving suffering while also providing comfort.[30] When nurses advocate for patients to receive effective pain management and are not heeded by providers, they may experience moral distress due to their powerlessness to adequately manage pain.[31,32] Similarly, when patient families are making the medical decisions and refusing the administration of pain medication despite the patient being in obvious pain, nurses may experience moral distress because they unable to gauge the patient's wishes and, therefore, feel as they are contributing to the patient's suffering.[33]

Another potential source of moral distress for nurses caring for patients at the end of life is iatrogenic pain. Iatrogenic pain is the pain derived by patients from their medical treatments. When care is deemed futile, the nurse may perceive treatment as an additional factor causing pain for their patient. This perception of futile care by the nurse may perpetuate moral distress. Green and colleagues'[34] study exploring the experiences of neonatal nurses found that nurses caring for neonates were able to cope with the infliction of pain on their patients when hope for recovery existed; however, once care was deemed futile, the neonatal nurses felt as they were torturing the neonate and experienced moral distress as a result. Nurses may also experience moral distress when patient families request painful treatments and interventions be implemented or attempted despite futility.[32] Additionally, in a systematic review exploring how professional nurses in a hospital experience moral distress,[35] futile care resulting in unwarranted pain and suffering among patients resulted in moral distress among nurses, especially when pediatric patients were involved.

When unable to effectively manage pain among patients with cancer, nurses may experience moral distress.[33,36,37] Given the nature of cancer as a disease, the sources of moral distress associated with pain management are similar to those related to end-of-life pain management. Researchers exploring moral distress and cancer pain management among oncology nurses in India found that the experience of moral distress was associated with perceived provision of futile care, inability to effectively advocate for pain and symptom management, interdisciplinary conflicts stemming from hierarchical structures within the organization, lack of resources to effectively manage pain and symptoms associated with cancer, and perceived powerlessness.[37]

DISCUSSION

The relationship between moral distress and pain management is not well explored within the critical care nursing literature. Despite this, there are implications to consider that may be applicable to critical care nurses based upon what is currently understood about pain management and moral distress within other nursing disciplines. Patients at the end of life and oncology patients are common patients encountered in the ICU because of their critical illnesses and conditions. Critical care nurses can empower themselves to care for patients receiving pain management where moral and ethical conflicts may arise by seeking education pertinent to pain management, attending pain management in services offered by their organizations, familiarizing themselves with pain management clinical practice guidelines, educating themselves on conditions which may predispose patients to pain, and participating in programs to support well-being through moral empowerment and resilience.

For moral distress precipitated by ethical and moral challenges associated with caring for patients at the end of life, palliative care education programs may be beneficial in reducing the moral distress. Nurses surveyed by De Brasi and colleagues[29] noted palliative care education programs need to be robust in order for them to effectively cope with moral distress experienced in their practice.[29] Similarly, programs to support nurses caring for patients with cancer should be both formally and informally designed to promote coping and resilience.[38] While it is imperative for nurses to take ownership of their own empowerment and resilience, organizations are also integral in equipping their nurses and other staff with the resources and skills to navigate the moral and ethical challenges of care.[38]

The National Academies of Science, Engineering, and Medicine's (NASEM) *The Future of Nursing 2020 to 2030*[39] calls for individual nurses, nurse leaders, and the systems in which they practice to institute strategies to support the well-being of nurses. NASEM calls for strategies to create programs focused on resilience and ethical competence which may also have implications for nurses caring for patients requiring pain management.[39] To address these strategies, organizations may consider providing moral distress consultation services,[4] ethics rounding,[40] Schwartz Center Rounds (structured forum for clinical and nonclinical staff to discuss emotional and social aspects of care related to a patient case),[41] moral resilience and mindfulness training,[42] formal debriefing processes,[43,44] empowerment programs,[45] and implementing strategies suggested within the American Association of Critical Care Nurses' Healthy Work Environment Framework.[46] For the development or sustainment of these programs, strategies to navigate the moral and ethical challenges associated with pain management should be incorporated.

SUMMARY

Critical care nurses experience several ethical and moral challenges in practice which may predispose them to the experience of moral distress. While the research surrounding moral distress resulting from pain management is limited and does not address critical care nurses specifically, critical care nurses caring for patients requiring pain management may encounter constraints when they are unable to effectively manage patient pain, especially among patients with cancer and patients at the end of life. Constraints noted within the literature include unclear goals of care, lack of support from organizations, powerlessness resulting from hierarchical structures between physicians and nurses, and family decisions overriding the judgment of nurses. Critical care nurses can empower themselves to cope with moral distress and advocate for their patients by educating themselves on evidence-based clinical practice guidelines regarding pain management, attending institution-developed in-services and programs regarding pain management, and accessing resources both within their organization and externally to promote well-being and resilience. To support critical care nurses and other health care professionals, organizations should consider developing programs to promote and support well-being. These programs should integrate moral and ethical challenges associated with pain management.

CLINICS CARE POINTS

- Critical care nurses may experience moral distress when they are unable to effectively manage pain.
- Challenges associated with pain management for patients at the end of life and oncology patients may precipitate moral distress.
- Care that is deemed futile or results in iatrogenic pain is a potential source of moral distress.
- Critical care nurses should familiarize themselves with current clinical practice guidelines regarding pain management such as those published by the SCCM.

DISCLOSURE

The author has no disclosures or conflicts of interest to report.

REFERENCES

1. Raja SN, Carr DB, Cohen M, et al. The revised International Association for the Study of Pain definition of pain: concepts, challenges, and compromises. Pain 2020;161(9):1976–82.
2. ANA Ethics Advisory Board. ANA position statement: the ethical responsibility to manage pain and the suffering it causes. OJIN: Online J Issues Nurs 2018;24(1).
3. Jameton A. Nursing practice: the ethical issues. Englewood Cliffs, NJ: Prentice-Hall; 1984.
4. Epstein EG, Shah R, Marshall MF. Effect of a moral distress consultation service on moral distress, empowerment, and a healthy work environment. HEC Forum 2021. https://doi.org/10.1007/s10730-021-09449-5.
5. Hamric AB. A case study of moral distress. J Hospice Palliat Nurs 2014;16(8): 457–63.
6. Jameton A. Dilemmas of moral distress: moral responsibility and nursing practice. AWHONNS Clin Issues Perinat Womens Health Nurs 1993;4(4):542–51.
7. Varcoe C, Pauly B, Webster G, et al. Moral distress: Tensions as springboards for action. HEC Forum 2012;24(1):51–62.
8. American Association of Critical Care Nurses, Recognize and address moral distress, Available at: https://www.aacn.org/~/media/aacn-website/clincial-resources/moral-distress/recognizing-addressing-moral-distress-quick-reference-guide.pdf. Accessed February 13, 2024.
9. Pavlish C, Brown-Saltzman K, So L, et al. Suppot: an evidence-based model for leaders addressing moral distress. J Nurs Adm 2016;46(6):313–20.
10. Dodek PM, Norena M, Ayas N, et al. Moral distress is associated with general workplace distress in intensive care unit personnel. J Crit Care 2019;50:122–5.
11. Karakachian A, Colbert A. Nurses' moral distress, burnout, and intentions to leave: an integrative review. J Forensic Nurs 2019;15(3):133–42.
12. Wolf AT, White KR, Epstein EG, et al. Palliative care and moral distress: an institutional survey of critical care nurses. Crit Care Nurse 2019;39(5):38–49.
13. Alimoradi Z, Jafari E, Lin CY, et al. Estimation of moral distress among nurses: a systematic review and meta-analysis. Nurs Ethics 2023;30(3):334–57.
14. Whitehead PB, Herbertson RK, Hamric AB, et al. Moral distress among healthcare professionals: report of an institution-wide survey. J Nurs Scholarsh 2015; 47(2):117–25.
15. Pota V, Coppolino F, Barbarisi A, et al. Pain in intensive care: a Narrative review. Pain Ther 2022;11(2):359–67.
16. Chanques G, Gélinas C. Monitoring pain in the intensive care unit (ICU). Intensive Care Med 2022;48(10):1508–11.
17. Puntillo KA, Max A, Timsit JF, et al. Determinants of procedural pain intensity in the intensive care unit. The Europain® study. Am J Respir Crit Care Med 2014; 189(1):39–47.
18. Devlin JW, Skrobik Y, Gélinas C, et al. Clinical practice guidelines for the prevention and management of pain, agitation/sedation, Delirium, immobility, and Sleep disruption in adult patients in the ICU. Crit Care Med 2018;46(9):e825–73.
19. Smith HAB, Besunder JB, Betters KA, et al. 2022 society of critical care medicine clinical practice guidelines on prevention and management of pain, agitation, neuromuscular blockade, and Delirium in critically ill pediatric patients with consideration of the ICU environment and early mobility. Pediatr Crit Care Med 2022;23(2):e74–110.

20. Ulrich BT, Lavandero R, Hart KA, et al. Critical care nurses' work environments: a baseline status report. Crit Care Nurse 2006;26(5):52–7, 46-50.

21. Ulrich BT, Lavandero R, Hart KA, et al. Critical care nurses' work environments 2008: a follow-up report. Crit Care Nurse 2009;29(2):93–102.

22. Ulrich BT, Lavandero R, Woods D, et al. Critical care nurse work environments 2013: a status report. Crit Care Nurse 2014;34(4):64–79.

23. Ulrich B, Barden C, Cassidy L, et al. Critical care nurse work environments 2018: findings and implications. Crit Care Nurse 2019;39(2):67–84.

24. Ulrich B, Cassidy L, Barden C, et al. National nurse work environments - october 2021: a status report. Crit Care Nurse 2022;42(5):58–70.

25. Miller PH, Epstein EG, Smith TB, et al. Critical care nurse leaders addressing moral distress: a qualitative study. Nurs Crit Care 2024. https://doi.org/10.1111/nicc.13045.

26. Tanaka Gutiez M, Efstathiou N, Innes R, et al. End-of-life care in the intensive care unit. Anaesthesia 2023;78(5):636–43.

27. Eddleman M, Montz K, Wocial LD. Moral distress in the ICU: measuring, tracking, and responding to staff experiences. Nurse Lead 2023;21(3):e64–72.

28. Bernhofer EI, Sorrell JM. Nurses managing patients' pain may experience moral distress. Clin Nurs Res 2015;24(4):401–14.

29. De Brasi EL, Giannetta N, Ercolani S, et al. Nurses' moral distress in end-of-life care: a qualitative study. Nurs Ethics 2021;28(5):614–27.

30. White D, Meeker MA. Guiding the process of dying: the personal impact on nurses. J Hosp Palliat Nurs 2019;21(5):390–6.

31. Ferrell BR. Understanding the moral distress of nurses witnessing medically futile care. Oncol Nurs Forum 2006;33(5):922–30.

32. Midtbust MH, Gjengedal E, Alnes RE. Moral distress - a threat to dementia care? A qualitative study of nursing staff members' experiences in long-term care facilities. BMC Health Serv Res 2022;22(1):290.

33. Pavlish C, Brown-Saltzman K, Hersh M, et al. Nursing priorities, actions, and regrets for ethical situations in clinical practice. J Nurs Scholarsh 2011;43(4):385–95.

34. Green J, Darbyshire P, Adams A, et al. It's agony for us as well: neonatal nurses reflect on iatrogenic pain. Nurs Ethics 2016;23(2):176–90.

35. Huffman DM, Rittenmeyer L. How professional nurses working in hospital environments experience moral distress: a systematic review. Crit Care Nurs Clin North Am 2012;24(1):91–100.

36. Buitrago J. Strategies to mitigate moral distress in oncology nursing. Clin J Oncol Nurs 2023;27(1):87–91.

37. LeBaron V, Beck SL, Black F, et al. Nurse moral distress and cancer pain management: an ethnography of oncology nurses in India. Cancer Nurs 2014;37(5):331–44.

38. Gillman L, Adams J, Kovac R, et al. Strategies to promote coping and resilience in oncology and palliative care nurses caring for adult patients with malignancy: a comprehensive systematic review. JBI Database System Rev Implement Rep 2015;13(5):131–204.

39. National Academies of Sciences, Engineering, and Medicine. The future of nursing 2020-2023: charting a path to achieve health equity. Washington, DC: The National Academies Press; 2021.

40. Chiafery MC, Hopkins P, Norton SA, Shaw MH. Nursing Ethics Huddles to Decrease Moral Distress among Nurses in the Intensive Care Unit. J Clin Ethics 2018;29(3):217–26.

41. Whitehead PB, Locklear TM, Carter KF. A longitudinal study of the impact of Schwartz center Rounds on moral distress. J Nurs Adm 2021;51(7–8):409–15.
42. Heinze KE, Hanson G, Holtz H, et al. Measuring health care interprofessionals' moral resilience: validation of the rushton moral resilience scale. J Palliat Med 2021;24(6):865–72.
43. Browning ED, Cruz JS. Reflective debriefing: a social work intervention addressing moral distress among ICU nurses. J Soc Work End-of-Life Palliat Care 2018; 14(1):44–72.
44. Morley G, Horsburgh CC. Reflective debriefs as a response to moral distress: two case study examples. HEC Forum 2021. https://doi.org/10.1007/s10730-021-09441-z.
45. Abbasi S, Ghafari S, Shahriari M, et al. Effect of moral empowerment program on moral distress in intensive care unit nurses. Nurs Ethics 2019;26(5):1494–504.
46. American Association of Critical Care Nurses. AACN standards for establishing and sustaining healthy work environments: a journey to excellence. 2 ed. American Association of Critical-Care Nurses 2016;14(3):187–97.

Management of Hip Fractures

Jeanne Morrison, PhD, MSN[a],*, Mary Morrison, BS[b]

KEYWORDS

- Hip fractures • Pain management • Risk factors • Surgery
- Preoperative and postoperative care • Rehabilitation

KEY POINTS

- The journey to recovery from a hip fracture can be daunting, with 11% becoming bedridden, 16% requiring admission to care facilities, and 80% needing a walking aid.
- Risk factors for hip fracture include age, sex, bone density, and certain medications can contribute to the likelihood of fractures.
- Various treatment options are examined, from conservative management to surgical interventions such as internal fixation and arthroplasty.

INTRODUCTION

Hip fractures represent a significant health challenge in the elderly population and are listed among the top 10 disabilities globally, with women accounting for 75% to 80% of these cases. In the United States alone, over 300,000 individuals suffer from hip fractures each year. The majority of these patients are around 80 year old, with women being more frequently affected than men. The mortality rates associated with hip fractures are alarming, with up to 10% of patients dying within 1 month and as high as 30% within 1 year.[1] Hip fractures are the leading cause of admission and hospitalization in orthopedic or trauma departments for people above 65 years. The financial burden is also substantial, with costs for fractures near the hip totaling 2 to 4 billion dollars annually.[2]

For survivors, the journey to recovery can be daunting, with 11% becoming bedridden, 16% requiring admission to care facilities, and 80% needing a walking aid. Hip fractures are categorized by their proximity to the hip capsule and the extent of displacement. This study focuses on 2 of the most prevalent types of hip fractures: femoral neck fracture (FNF; intracapsular), accounting for 45% to 53%, and intertrochanteric fractures (extracapsular), constituting 38% to 50% of all hip fractures.[1]

[a] College of Nursing, Walden University, 100 Washington Avenue South, Suite 1210, Minneapolis, MN 55401, USA; [b] College of Psychology Doctoral Program, Walden University, 100 Washington Avenue South, Suite 1210, Minneapolis, MN, USA
* Corresponding author.
E-mail address: Jeanne.morrison@mail.waldenu.edu

Crit Care Nurs Clin N Am 36 (2024) 575–584
https://doi.org/10.1016/j.cnc.2024.04.007

RISK FACTORS

Certain factors can increase a person's risk of hip fracture. Some of these factors are immutable, while others can be influenced to help mitigate the risk. Unchangeable risk factors include age, particularly for women over 85 years, who are 10 times more likely to experience a hip fracture than those in their 60s. Women are more affected than men, with men having half the estimated risk.[1] Previous fractures, lower socioeconomic status, and specific conditions such as bone diseases or cancers contribute to risk and cannot be altered.[2]

Elleby and colleagues explored the link between self-reported health and mobility and the risk of hip fractures over 35 years. Participants included 16,536 men and women aged between 26 and 65 years. The research provided insights into predicting long-term hip fracture risks based on early self-reported physical health data. It emphasizes a specific period in mid-life as crucial for using health questions to pinpoint individuals at an increased risk for fragility fractures. The findings advocate for incorporating this knowledge into risk prediction tools and preventive strategies during one's middle years, underlining the significance of early detection and prevention for those at heightened risk of hip fractures.[3]

Falls, the primary cause of up to 90% of hip fractures, can be minimized.[4] Factors such as low body weight, malnutrition, or bone density, often linked to osteoporosis, increase risk, yet staying active and good nutrition can counteract this since exercise fortifies bones (W.A. Morrison, MD, orthopedic surgeon, personal communication, February 14, 2024).

Medications may elevate risk by reducing bone density or causing side effects such as dizziness, potentially leading to falls. Such medications include steroids, certain thyroid and stomach acid drugs, water pills, and blood pressure medications. Additionally, antidepressants, anxiety medications, and painkillers can induce drowsiness or instability, which may increase falling.[1,5,6]

PRESENTATION

Patients with a fractured hip experience considerable pain in the hip and groin area and typically cannot walk. The injured leg may appear shorter if the fracture is displaced. They are usually transported to the emergency room, where a radiograph confirms the fracture location. Treatment generally involves pain management and often necessitates surgical intervention to treat the fracture. Medical evaluation is crucial, especially if the patient has other health issues or a chance of head injury, which is common in falls. The patient's health, history, mobility, and cognitive state are all reviewed to decide the best surgical approach and anticipate how they might recover.[1]

DIAGNOSIS

Patients with hip injuries usually report anterior groin pain that radiates to the thigh or buttock and have trouble bearing weight on the affected leg following a fall or trauma. Physical examination may reveal various signs, including hip deformity, external rotation, abduction, or shortening of the affected leg, tenderness in the groin and anterior hip, pain during the log roll maneuver (gentle rotation of the lower leg and thigh), or unable to raise a straight leg while lying on the back. Ecchymosis (bruising) is generally not present initially. It is also essential to assess the neurovascular status of the affected limb, checking distal pulses and sensations.[1]

For diagnosing hip fractures, the first steps are typically cross-table lateral hip and anteroposterior pelvis radiographs.[7] MRI may be used if a fracture is still suspected despite negative radiographs.[1]

According to an orthopedic surgeon (W.A. Morrison, MD, February 2024), the treatment of hip fractures differs because of the blood supply to the hip. The blood supply to the femoral head and neck is precarious, so if there is a displaced fracture, the blood supply is cut off, and the bone dies, resulting in avascular necrosis. If the fracture to the femoral neck is not displaced, then the blood supply may be intact so that treatment with displaced and nondisplaced fractures is different.

Types of Fractures

Intertrochanteric fracture

An intertrochanteric fracture occurs between the greater and lesser trochanter, 2 prominent bony points on the femur (thigh bone) near the hip joint. While they can result from high-impact incidents such as vehicle accidents or falls in younger individuals, they predominantly occur in older adults due to osteoporosis (bone weakening) associated with aging. Moreover, it can significantly impair mobility and independence. Even a fall from standing height can lead to such a fracture for older adults. Reports from the US Centers for Disease Control and Prevention indicate that hip fractures lead to hospitalization for over 300,000 individuals annually.[8]

An intertrochanteric fracture can range from a simple break with the bone pieces well aligned (stable fracture). However, even with this type of fracture, prolonged immobility carries its risks, especially in the elderly.[1,4,8]

According to an orthopedic surgeon (W.A. Morrison, MD, personal communication, February 2024), intertrochanteric fractures are either nondisplaced or displaced, but all require surgical intervention to stabilize and mobilize the patient. Surgical intervention may involve the placement of a metal implant to maintain the correct alignment and stabilization of the fractured bone during healing. Metal screws, plates, and/or rods are used to hold the bone fragments in place until they heal. An *intramedullary hip compression screw* is a device used for the internal fixation of certain types of hip fractures, especially intertrochanteric regions or FNFs. These screws are designed to be inserted into the medullary canal of the femur, the inner, hollow portion of the thigh bone. The device aims to stabilize the fracture, promote proper alignment and healing, and allow early patient mobilization. The design typically involves a large screw (the compression screw) that is threaded through the femoral head and neck, capturing the fracture fragments. This is often done in conjunction with a plate or nail (the intramedullary nail) that runs down the shaft of the femur, providing additional stability and distributing the load along the length of the bone. The "compression" part of the name comes from the device ability to apply a compressive force across the fracture site, which helps the healing process by increasing the contact and stability between the broken bone ends.

This method of fixation is particularly advantageous for elderly patients with osteoporotic bone, where other types of fixations might not provide sufficient stability, and in situations where the anatomy or the type of fracture makes other surgical options less feasible. The goal of using an intramedullary hip compression screw is to achieve a stable fixation that allows the bone to heal in a proper position while minimizing the risk of complications such as nonunion.[1,5]

Femoral neck fractures

FNFs represent a distinct category of hip fractures. This region, the femoral neck, serves as the connecting structure between the femoral shaft and the femoral head. The interaction of the femoral head and the acetabulum forms the hip joint. Owing to its position at the junction, the femoral neck is susceptible to fractures (W.A. Morrison, MD, orthopedic surgeon, personal communication, February 14, 2024).

FNFs have a high incidence of severe health complications, particularly among older women. Treatment should be initiated promptly with surgical intervention and comprehensive multidisciplinary perioperative care. Treatment options may include open reduction internal fixation, hemiarthroplasty (HA), and total hip arthroplasty (THA), each with its advantages and disadvantages. Timely surgical intervention is crucial as delays are associated with increased mortality and complications.[5-7]

Surgery options vary, and the choice depends on the fracture type and the patient's age, health, and mental state. Timing is crucial; delays can lead to increased pain, anxiety, and poor recovery outcomes.[5,7] An orthopedic surgeon (W.A. Morrison, MD, February 14, 2024) states that the treatment of hip fractures differs because of the blood supply to the hip. The blood supply to the femoral head and neck is precarious, so if there is a displaced fracture, the blood supply is cut off and the bone dies, resulting in avascular necrosis. If the fracture to the femoral neck is not displaced, then the blood supply may be intact so that treatment with displaced and nondisplaced fractures is different.

Typically, internal fixation is the preferred treatment of patients with nondisplaced fractures of the femoral neck. Displaced FNFs in younger patients are often treated with closed reduction and pinning to avoid hip replacement.[1] However, this has a risk of avascular necrosis (bone tissue death due to the lack of blood supply). Patients older than 65 years with displaced FNF usually undergo hemi or total arthroplasty (joint replacement; W.A. Morrison, MD, orthopedic surgeon, personal communication, February 14, 2024).

The prevailing data endorse the application of internal fixation, utilizing either cannulated or partially threaded screws, for treating a majority of patients with nondisplaced FNF. These techniques typically yield favorable results regarding pain relief and hip functionality.[5] Nevertheless, the increased likelihood of needing subsequent surgeries with internal fixation because of avascular necrosis or nonunion means that arthroplasty might be a better option for patients with displaced FNF (W.A. Morrison, MD, orthopedic surgeon, personal communication, February 14, 2024).

For displaced FNF in older individuals, the debate over choosing internal fixation versus arthroplasty has primarily settled, leaning toward arthroplasty as the more effective approach for most such fractures. However, the decision between HA, THA, and cement application must still be clearly defined. THA, potentially more fitting for active patients due to its enhanced postsurgical performance and implant durability, contrasts with HA, which might be adequate for patients with extensive comorbidities who are less capable of enduring longer surgeries or the prospect of additional surgeries.[5] Moreover, integrating THA with dual mobility cups may mitigate and lessen the dislocation risks commonly associated with standard THA. Despite inconclusive evidence, the preference for THA is rising globally (W.A. Morrison, MD, orthopedic surgeon, personal communication, February 14, 2024).

Although studies indicate superior functional outcomes and a reduced need for revision surgeries with cemented arthroplasty compared to its uncemented counterpart, the global trend is shifting toward using uncemented components. Cemented arthroplasty poses the additional threat of bone cement implantation syndrome (BCIS). BCIS is a complication causing cardiovascular instability and possibly severe reactions such as hypotension or cardiac arrest.[5] Prompt detection and treatment of BCIS with aggressive fluid management, inotropic support, and pulmonary vasodilators can be effective.[5]

Treatment

Preoperative
Treatment for a fractured hip generally involves pain management. Before surgery, thorough medical evaluation is crucial, especially if the patient has other health issues or a

chance of head injury, which is common in falls.[1] For diagnosis, the first steps are typically cross-table lateral hip and anteroposterior pelvis radiographs. A computed axial tomography scan and/or MRI may be used if a fracture is still suspected despite negative X-rays.[1]

The patient's health, history, mobility, and cognitive state are all reviewed to decide the best surgical approach and anticipate how they might recover.[5] Patients with hip fractures often face other health issues, making extensive, team-based care critical. The patient's health, history, mobility, and cognitive state are all reviewed to decide the best surgical approach and anticipate how they might recover. Upon arriving at the hospital, patients receive intravenous (IV) de fluids to combat fluid or blood loss and electrolyte imbalances.[5,8] Managing pain properly is essential but must be done cautiously to avoid side effects such as delirium.[5] According to the orthopedic surgeon (W.A. Morrison, MD, personal communication, February 2024) also obtain an electrocardiogram (EKG), chest radiograph, complete blood count (CBC), electrolytes, renal function studies, and type and screening for blood type.

The American Academy of Orthopedic Surgeons recommends that surgery ideally occurs within 24 to 48 hours of the injury unless other health issues must first be stabilized.[9] Early surgery helps control pain, shortens hospital stays, and reduces complications. However, there is a significant rate of postoperative complications, both systemic (such as myocardial infarction and deep vein thrombosis) and surgical (such as wound infections). Complications can lead to severe outcomes, including loss of mobility, independence, or death. Many studies have identified predictive factors for perioperative complications, including gender, age, comorbidities, and physical status at the time of injury.[2] The time-to-surgery interval is controversial, with studies presenting varied findings on the relationship between surgery timing and complication rates. While some guidelines recommend surgery within 24 hours of injury, others suggest a 48 hour window, and there is no international consensus on the optimal timing.[2] Although surgery within 6 hours does not necessarily lower mortality rates, it decreases perioperative complications, allows for faster postoperative recovery, and shortens the time to hospital discharge. Waiting for more than 24 hours for surgery is linked to increased mortality within 30 days. The choice of procedure depends on the specific case and is determined by the surgeon.[1,2,9]

Perioperative management techniques
Antibiotics. Before and after surgery (specifically 1–2 hours before and 24 hours after), doctors recommend antibiotics to prevent infections in the joint.[1]

Anesthesia. During surgery, either spinal or general anesthesia is used to prevent pain. In addition to the main anesthesia, nerve blocks can relieve extra pain and improve overall recovery.[1]

Venous thromboembolism prophylaxis. Patients with a hip fracture are more likely to develop blood clots due to not moving much (immobility). To prevent this, doctors recommend using medication (chemoprophylaxis) rather than just physical methods to prevent clotting (mechanical prophylaxis).[1]

Transfusion. After surgery, if a patient's hemoglobin (a protein in red blood cells) level is very low (<7 g per dL) and no specific heart-related risks exist, a blood transfusion might be necessary to replace lost blood.[1]

Postoperative Care

Pain management
Effective pain management and preventive measures are essential postsurgery.[8] The risk of another fracture is real, so strategies such as medication and lifestyle changes

are vital to prevent further issues. Complications such as infections, joint issues, and blood clots can occur. Postoperative care should include aggressive pain management, venous thromboembolism prophylaxis, and interventions to reduce perioperative delirium and complications.[5] A team of various health care professionals, including nurses, orthopedic surgeons, hospitalists, dietitians, geriatric services, social workers, and physical and occupational therapists, work together to reduce complications and deaths during the hospital stay and improve the patient's ability to function after surgery.[1]

Starting rehabilitation and weight-bearing activities within 24 hours after surgery are linked to better mobility outcomes.[7] After leaving the hospital, the patient might continue rehabilitation as an inpatient at home or outpatient, depending on their needs. Physical therapists are crucial in customizing and guiding the rehabilitation process.[1] Postsurgery patients may require mobility aids such as walkers or crutches. Weight-bearing on the affected hip is generally directed by the surgeon. Some patients might need to stay in a rehabilitation facility until they regain strength and mobility. The postoperative period also involves proactive measures to prevent complications such as pneumonia, bedsores, or blood clots and includes exercises to maintain leg function.[1]

Long-term postsurgery, some patients may experience a limp, fatigue, or stiffness in the hip, which physical therapy can help alleviate. In rare cases, there may be discomfort from the metal implants or complications such as nonhealing fractures or infections, potentially requiring further surgery.[1]

Medications

Hip fractures are associated with significant pain, which may necessitate the use of opioids. Owing to the high potential for addiction associated with opioids, close monitoring of patients for early signs of dependence is crucial. Health care professionals should prescribe these drugs in a manner that is clinically appropriate and complies with regulatory guidelines. Other types of pain management tools may be used as well.[10]

Opioids

Hereford and colleagues focused on opioid usage following THA. The study hypothesizes that a notable portion of elderly patients who have never used opioids before may start using them chronically after undergoing surgery for hip fractures. The study included 219 patients who had hip fractures between 2016 and 2019. Opioid usage was tracked using the state's prescription monitoring program. The study found that 26% (58 patients) became chronic users of opioids after their surgery. Specifically, among the 188 patients who had never used opioids before the surgery, 23% (43 patients) started using opioids chronically after their hip fracture surgery. Among the 31 patients who were already using opioids before their surgery, nearly half (48% or 15 patients) continued to use opioids chronically after the surgery. Patients who became chronic users after surgery were more likely to be white, younger, and were already using opioids before their surgery. The type of surgery (arthroplasty vs fixation) did not significantly affect the likelihood of chronic opioid use. Chronic opioid use after surgery for hip fracture in elderly patients is surprisingly common, with about 23% of patients who had never used opioids before becoming chronic users after their surgery. The study underscores the importance of careful monitoring and regulation of postoperative narcotic prescriptions by orthopedic surgeons to prevent prolonged usage. Hereford and colleagues posit a gap in research about opioid use in elderly patients post-hip fracture surgery.[10]

Morphine and analgesics

Rapeepat and colleagues' retrospective study analyzed hip fracture treatment outcomes by comparing intravenous morphine with other analgesics. It involved 1531 patients, focusing on postoperative pain, hospitalization costs, and adverse effects. In this study, nearly two-thirds of patients received analgesics as needed, while over a third had them prescribed preemptively. Intravenous morphine was the favored choice in both groups, with the intravenous (IV) group's costs slightly higher at $2277, compared to $2174 for other analgesics. The group using alternative analgesics used more acetaminophen and selective non-steroidal anti-inflammatory drugs (NSAIDs). Pain levels were comparable between the groups, yet those on IV morphine reported more stomach and intestinal side effects at a rate of 24% versus 10.5%. The research found no significant difference in pain scores between groups, but the IV morphine group incurred higher hospital costs and experienced more gastrointestinal side effects, primarily constipation. The study underscores the impact of analgesic choice on medical expenses and hospitalization outcomes, advocating for further research in diverse settings.[11]

Nerve blocks

Davis and colleagues' research analyzed the effect of different anesthesia types on pain and opioid use after hip surgeries. The study included 588 patients and found that peripheral nerve block (PNB) reduced opioid needs early on but might increase certain complications such as delirium. While PNB was effective in managing pain with less opioid use, the study advised further investigation into its link with specific postoperative issues.[1,5,12]

The Department of Orthopedic Surgery aimed to compare the effects of PNB and local infiltration analgesia (LIA) on opioid consumption in the early postoperative period for patients with hip fracture. The median age of the patient was 82 years, with 67% being female. The PNB group was significantly less likely to use opioids at 24 and 48 hours postoperatively compared to the general anesthesia (GA) group. However, patients with a length of stay (LOS) of 10 days or more were more likely to require opioids within the first 24 and 48 hour postsurgery. Postoperative delirium (POD) was the most common complication. Patients in the PNB group had a higher likelihood of experiencing any complications compared to those in the GA group. There was no significant difference in complication rates when comparing the LIA and GA groups. The study concludes that while PNB can effectively reduce the need for opioids after hip fracture surgery, it does not necessarily mitigate the risk of postoperative complications such as delirium.[13]

Pain management tool

Shen and colleagues explored a new preoperative pain management model using instant messaging software for elderly patients with hip fracture. It was a randomized controlled trial with 100 participants over 65 years, split into test and control groups. The methodology involved a comprehensive pain management approach, including early fascia iliaca compartment block (FICB) and closed-loop pain management. The results indicated that the test group had quicker FICB completion, better pain control, and higher analgesic satisfaction. The study concluded that the new model improved the timeliness and effectiveness of analgesia, though it recommended more extensive future studies to confirm the effects on POD. The new pain management mode, supported by instant messaging and multidisciplinary cooperation, significantly improved the timeliness and effectiveness of analgesia for elderly patients with hip fractures. It allowed for FICB to be completed sooner and improved overall pain management.[14]

Cognitive

Cadel and colleagues review the rehabilitation methods for adults with hip fractures and cognitive impairment, summarizing 17 studies. It underscores the need for more research on personal and family experiences and customizing interventions for cognitive challenges. The recommendations stress the importance of understanding these experiences, personalizing treatments, and ensuring long-term, collaborative care strategies. In assisting those with cognitive impairment, a comprehensive approach is critical. This includes a nurturing environment, regular mental and physical exercise, social engagement, and a stable routine with proper nutrition and sleep. Personalizing activities and ongoing dialogue with health care professionals are vital for adequate care and adaptation as needs change.[15]

Cadel and colleagues emphasize the critical need for personalized and family-centered approaches in rehabilitating adults with hip fractures and cognitive issues. It calls for research into personal experiences and tailored care strategies. Caring for those with cognitive challenges requires a holistic strategy, including a supportive setting, balanced routines, and open communication with health care professionals, ensuring care evolves with individual needs.[15]

Pfeiffer and colleagues' study evaluated a cognitive behavioral therapy program aimed at reducing fall-related anxiety and enhancing rehabilitation outcomes for the elderly. The research included 115 individuals, with an average age of 82.5, years predominantly women (70%), who had experienced hip or pelvic fractures and were undergoing geriatric inpatient rehabilitation. Participants were split into 2 groups: a control group receiving standard care and an intervention group (Rehab + I) that received 8 extra sessions, a home visit, and 4 follow-up calls over 2 months postdischarge, along with relaxation and meaningful activities and setting mobility goals. The results showed improvements in psychological well-being and physical performance for the intervention group but no increase in daily walking time. The investigators suggest more research on a less intensive intervention that may still be beneficial during the inpatient phase.[16]

Prevention/Intervention

Bone mineral density

Low bone mineral density (BMD) is a significant risk factor for hip fractures. To address this

1. *Postoperative care:* Patients should be assessed for osteoporosis and treated accordingly. Often, oral bisphosphonates after surgery are recommended.[17]
2. *Long-term treatment:* Those with low BMD should receive long-term treatment with medications such as bisphosphonates,[5] parathyroid analogs (eg, teriparatide or abaloparatide), or receptive activator of nuclear factor kappa-B lagand (RANKL inhibitors) (eg, denosumab or romosozumab).[18]
3. *Vitamin D:* It is essential to check vitamin D levels, especially in individuals over 65 years. Low levels are linked to weak muscles, low BMD, and a higher risk of hip fractures.[1]

Physical activity and exercise

Being physically active is crucial for preventing first-time and repeat hip fractures.[19] This includes low to moderate aerobic exercise, resistance, strength, and proprioceptive (balance and position awareness) training. It not only reduces osteoporosis and improves hip function and life quality but also cuts the risk of injuries from falls by up to 40%.[1] Practicing tai chi, which involves strength and balance training, can reduce the rate of injurious falls by half.[1]

SUMMARY

In conclusion, managing hip fractures in women involves a detailed, patient-specific approach. It requires a coordinated team, timely intervention, and thorough postoperative care to ensure the best possible recovery and quality of life.[2] Our understanding of risk factors such as age, sex, bone density, and medication effects on fracture likelihood must inform our preventative strategies and treatment regimens. As this article has examined, the interplay between conservative and surgical management options, the use of perioperative care to reduce complications, and the innovative approaches to pain management represent the current state of care. Looking ahead, it is evident that continued research into pain management, surgical techniques, and postoperative rehabilitation is essential. The ultimate goal remains to not only extend life but to enhance the quality of life, minimizing pain and maximizing function and independence for women suffering from hip fractures.

CLINICS CARE POINTS

- A collaborative multidisciplinary team approach is essential in managing complex cases such as hip fractures.
- The treatment of hip fractures differs because of the blood supply to the hip. The blood supply to the femoral head and neck is precarious, so if there is a displaced fracture, the blood supply is cut off and the bone dies, resulting in avascular necrosis.
- Effective postoperative care, including pain control and bone density preservation, is crucial for mitigating future hip fracture risks.

REFERENCES

1. Schroeder JD, Turner SP, Buck E. Hip fractures: diagnosis and management. Am Fam Physician 2022;106(6):675–83. Available at: https://search.ebscohost.com/login.aspx?direct=true&AuthType=shib&db=mnh&AN=36521464&site=eds-live&scope=site. Accessed January 2024.
2. Daginnus A, Schmitt J, Graw JA, et al. Rate of complications after hip fractures caused by prolonged time-to-surgery depends on the patient's individual type of fracture and its Treatment. J Pers Med 2023;13(10). https://doi.org/10.3390/jpm13101470.
3. Elleby C, Skott P, Johansson S-E, et al. Long-term association of hip fractures with questions of physical health in a cohort of men and women. PLoS One 2023;17(3):e0283564.
4. Doro C. Intertrochanteric fracture. OTA Int. Available at: https://ota.org/for-patients/find-info-body-part/3720#/+/0/score,date_na_dt/desc/. Accessed January 18, 2024.
5. Sekeitto AR, Sikhauli N, van der Jagt DR, et al. The management of displaced femoral neck fractures: a narrative review. EFORT Open Rev 2021;6(2):139–44.
6. Holly C, Rittenmeyer L, Weeks SM. Evidence-based clinical audit criteria for the prevention and management of delirium in the postoperative patient with a hip fracture. Orthop Nurs 2014;33(1):27–34.
7. Florschutz AV, Langford JR, Haidukewych GJ, et al. Femoral neck fractures: current management. J Orthop Trauma 2015;29(3):121–9.

8. Center for Disease Control and Prevention. Injury prevention and control: keep on your feet-preventing older adult falls. Available at: https://www.cdc.gov/injury/features/older-adult-falls/index.html. Accessed January 20, 2024.

9. American Academy of Orthopaedic Surgeons. Management of hip fractures in older adults: evidence-based clinical practice guidelines. 2021. Available at: https://www.aaos.org/hipfxcpg. Accessed February 1, 2024.

10. Hereford TE, Porter A, Stambough JB, et al. Prevalence of chronic opioid use in the elderly after hip fracture surgery. J Arthroplasty 2022;37(7):S530–5.

11. Rapeepat S, Phichayut P, Krittai T, et al. Outcomes of hip fracture treatment with intravenous morphine and with other analgesics: postoperative analgesic medical expense, severity of pain and hospitalisation—a retrospective study. J Orthop Surg Res 2023;18(1):1–10.

12. Davis JM, Cuadra M, Roomian T, et al. Impact of anesthesia selection on post-op pain management in operatively treated hip fractures. Injury 2023;54(8). https://doi.org/10.1016/j.injury.2023.110872.

13. Department of Orthopedic Surgery. Update understanding of opioids: impact of anesthesia selection on post-op pain management in operatively treated hip fractures. Mental Health Weekly Digest. September 2023. Available at: https://search.ebscohost.com/login.aspx?db=edsgea&AN=edsgcl.764504630. Accessed February 2024.

14. Shen Y, Liu W, Zhu Z, et al. Application of a preoperative pain management mode based on instant messaging software in elderly hip fracture patients: a randomized controlled trial. BMC Geriatr 2023;23(1):186.

15. Cadel L, Kuluski K, Wodchis WP, et al. Rehabilitation interventions for persons with hip fracture and cognitive impairment: a scoping review. PLoS One 2022;17(8):e0273038.

16. Pfeiffer K, Kampe K, Klenk J, et al. Effects of an intervention to reduce fear of falling and increase physical activity during hip and pelvic fracture rehabilitation. Age Ageing 2020;49(5):771–8.

17. Schroeder JD, Turner SP, Buck E. Hip fractures. Am Fam Physician 2022;106(6):675–83. Available at: https://www.aafp.org/pubs/afp/issues/2022/1200/hip-fractures.html. Accessed February 2, 2024.

18. American College of Obstetricians and Gynecologists. Osteoporosis treatment: Updated guidelines from ACOG. Am Fam Physician 2023;108(1):100–4. Available at: https://www.aafp.org/pubs/afp/issues/2023/0700/practice-guidelines-osteoporosis-treatment.html. Accessed February 2, 2024.

19. Akan I, Bacaksiz T. Risk factors for hip fracture after simple fall in the elderly population. Eurasian Journal of Medical Investigation 2023;7(4):373–7.

Chronic Postsurgical Pain

Steven Wooden, DNP, CRNA, NSPM-C*

KEYWORDS

- Chronic pain • Postsurgical pain • Pain • Chronic postsurgical pain • CPSP

KEY POINTS

- Chronic pain is a devastating condition, emotionally, physically, economically, and socially.
- Chronic pain caused by surgical intervention is often ignored.
- Chronic postsurgical pain risks can be reduced.
- Chronic postsurgical pain is difficult to treat.

INTRODUCTION

It is estimated that 20.9% of US adults (51.6 million persons) experienced chronic pain, and 6.9% (17.1 million persons) experienced debilitating, life-altering chronic pain that results in substantial restrictions to daily activities.[1] Chronic pain is generally defined as persistent or recurrent pain lasting longer than 3 months and is classified by the World Health Organization's International Classification of Diseases (ICD) into 7 categories. They are primary, postsurgical, headache, musculoskeletal, cancer, neuropathic, and visceral pain.[2]

Among those, chronic postsurgical pain (CPSP) is likely the most frustrating chronic pain to deal with because it is the result of a surgical procedure that is intended to improve a person's health rather than create a new problem. In addition, surgical procedures that result in chronic pain are often caused by damage to a nerve, which can cause severe neuropathic symptoms often impacting the quality of life more than a nonneuropathic chronic pain.[3,4]

Compounding the problem of CPSP is the widespread marginalization of patients with chronic pain by health care providers.[5] There are often implicit biases and unmet expectations concerning the outcomes of a surgical procedure that contribute to this marginalization. In addition, health care education in the identification and treatment of CPSP is often lacking in both medicine and nursing.

Nurses are in an excellent position to help patients who are at high risk of developing CPSP, identify patients who might have CPSP, and recommend as well as implement

Texas Christian University, 2800 West Bowie Street, Fort Worth, TX 76109, USA
* 365 Ling Street, Bayou Vista, TX 77563.
E-mail address: S.Wooden@TCU.edu

Crit Care Nurs Clin N Am 36 (2024) 585–595
https://doi.org/10.1016/j.cnc.2024.04.008
0899-5885/24/© 2024 Elsevier Inc. All rights reserved.

treatment options that are based on nursing theory. A holistic approach for the treatment of CPSP lead by nurses is often the best approach for this complex problem.[6]

DISCUSSION
What Is Chronic Pain?

To properly identify CPSP and create an effective treatment plan, it is important to understand the value of pain and the pathologic nature of chronic pain. Pain is critical for survival. In the short term, pain notifies us of potential tissue damage and encourages us to react to prevent additional harm.[7]

In general, there are 2 types of peripheral pain. Pain that originates from nerve trauma called neuropathic pain, and pain that originates from tissue trauma called nociceptive pain. Most chronic pain is a mixed state of neuropathic and nociceptive pain that becomes centralized and pathologic.

During the normal process of pain perception and response, there are 4 actions that occur. Those actions are transduction, transmission, modulation, and perception (**Table 1**). They are all critical in the normal human response to painful stimulation.[8]

1. *Transduction*: Stimulation of tissue beyond a certain threshold, which then activates nerve endings.
2. *Transmission:* Information about stimulation that is carried from the site of stimulation or injury to the brain through central spinothalamic pathways.
3. *Modulation:* Various sites along the central pathway serve to either reduce or modify the information about the stimulation. These inhibitory mechanisms are important in reducing constant stimulation in the central nervous system, allowing only potentially harmful information to reach the brain. Occasionally the information is enhanced, but normally it is inhibited.
4. *Perception:* The forebrain of the human processes the information and creates a subjective awareness useful in avoiding future injuries and understanding the nature of the problem.

The process incorporates a number of receptors and chemical mediators that are important in normal pain processing.

Pain unabated over time may alter pain pathways, resulting in central sensitization and impairment to the central nervous system. Several changes take place within 3 areas of the body during the transition from acute to chronic pain.[9]

1. In the periphery, the pain threshold is reduced because of a prolonged inflammatory response. The activation of lymphocytes and the release of inflammatory material such as interleukins, substance P, and calcitonin gene-related peptide leads to peripheral sensitization.
2. Within the spinal cord, chronic stimulation creates an increase in nerve pathways that promote hyperexcitability. Normally dormant receptors such as N-methyl-D-

Table 1	
Components of the pain process	
Process	**Purpose**
Transduction	Site of painful stimulation
Transmission	Pain information from stimulus carried to the brain
Modulation	Modification of pain information, usually inhibition
Perception	Subjective awareness

aspartate (NMDA) become stimulated by an influx of magnesium leading to a condition called "wind-up." Wind-up creates an enhanced sensation to stimulation called allodynia. The combination of these complex neuroplastic activities creates a pathologic combination of a reduced stimulation threshold with escalating neuronal activity in the dorsal horn of the spinal cord called "central sensitization".
3. Often overlooked is the impact these changes have on the brain. There is a strong correlation between chronic pain and changes to mental status that leads to maladaptive pain coping ability, anxiety, and depression.

Chronic pain creates a number of pathologic conditions that are difficult to treat. Among the symptoms of chronic pain are hyperalgesia, allodynia, widespread pain, and sleep disorders. *Hyperalgesia* is an intensification of pain due to reduction in modulation. As an example, a patient may appear to have an exaggerated response to the inflation of the blood pressure cuff. *Allodynia* is a conversion of normally nonpainful stimulation to intensely painful stimulation. Patients may indicate that a soft touch or the movement of bed sheets causes intense localized pain. *Widespread pain* often accompanies the development of chronic pain. Incisional pain may be reported well beyond the expected area of injury. *Sleep disorders* are very common with chronic pain. Lack of sleep diminishes the body's ability to modulate pain and creates other issues such as fatigue, memory loss, and irritability.

What Is Chronic Postsurgical Pain and How Do We Identify It?

Some degree of acute pain is expected after a surgical procedure because of the physiologic response to tissue damage after an incision. This discomfort, no matter how it is treated, is expected to pass as a normal part of the healing process. However, as many as 33% of those undergoing common surgical procedures report persist or intermittent pain at 1 year postsurgical procedure.[10]

Many patients have pain preoperatively, and this can complicate the diagnosis of CPSP. Most researchers agree that a diagnosis of CPSP can be made when all of the following conditions are met[11]

1. The pain is persistent or recurrent and has lasted longer than 3 months postsurgical procedure.
2. The pain began or increased in intensity after a surgical procedure.
3. The pain is primarily located in the area of the surgical procedure.
4. The pain cannot be attributed to an infection, a malignancy, a pre-existing pain condition, or any other condition.

One of the compounding problems with this diagnosis is that the condition is usually not identified until months have passed and the neuroplastic activity associated with chronic pain has begun. This makes CPSP at this point difficult to treat. For that reason, it is very important to identify those at risk prior to surgery, implement preventative measures for those at risk, and begin treatment as soon as possible for those who develop symptoms of CPSP (**Table 2**).

OBSERVATION/ASSESSMENT/EVALUATION

Predictors of CPSP can help to isolate likely candidates. When preparing patients for surgery, it is important to identify risk factors and plan accordingly. Some of the more common risk factors for CPSP that may be difficult or impossible to alter are female sex, younger age, obesity, preoperative pain regardless of the site, and specific surgical procedures. Other factors that can and should be addressed and modified prior to surgery are anxiety, depression, catastrophizing, and generalized stress.

Table 2 Incidences of chronic postsurgical pain[a] adapted from multiple studies[36]			
Abdominal surgery	17%–21%	Inguinal hernia repair	5%–63%
Amputation	30%–85%	Knee arthroplasty	13%–44%
Cesarean section	6%–65%	Mastectomy	11%–57%
Cholecystectomy	3%–56%	Sternotomy	7%–50%
Craniotomy	7%–65%	Thoracotomy	5%–71%
Hip arthroplasty	7%–23%	—	—

[a] The definition of CPSP from the ICD, 11th Revision.

A study conducted in 2020 identified 6 factors that could reliably predict the risk of CPSP with a 70% success rate, allowing for a more tailored surgical and anesthesia approach to reduce the risk of CPSP development in those patients. Those predicting factors were type of surgical procedure, young age, diminished physical health for age, mental health issues, preoperative pain in the surgical field, and preoperative pain in other areas.[12]

CONTROVERSIAL ISSUES

Some studies suggest that smoking may have a link to CPSP. This issue is complicated by the fact that nicotine is an analgesic. Thoracic surgery is a common procedure for smokers due to the higher incidence of pulmonary diseases among smokers. Studies found that those who continued to smoke after procedure had a lower incidence of CPSP than those who quit, but the study authors also cautioned against encouraging smoking to reduce the incidence of CPSP. The link between smokers and reports of increased CPSP appears to be related to the effort to stop smoking postsurgery.[13]

Preoperative opioid use has also been linked to a higher incidence of CPSP. It is unclear as to whether CPSP is caused by opioid use, or if the use of opioids is a result of chronic pain. There is a link between opioid metabolites and opioid-induced hyperalgesia (OIH) in those with long-term opioid use.[14] This is the basis for considering preoperative opioid use as a risk factor for CPSP. One of the main risk factors associated with CPSP is preoperative pain. For those using opioids to treat the preoperative pain, the likelihood of developing CPSP appears to escalate.[15]

Addressing the Preoperative Risk Factors

Even those risk factors that cannot be changed will help identify patients at risk when considering all the other factors (**Table 3**). Doing so will help providers look for modifications that might help mitigate the risks of CPSP development.

Table 3 Risk factors for chronic postsurgical pain	
Factor	Conditions the Promote CPSP
Surgery type	See **Box 1**
Anesthesia type	Regional anesthesia reduces risk while inhalation anesthesia enhances the risk
Preoperative pain	Pain at the surgery site or anywhere on the body increases risk
Mental health	Depression and anxiety increase risk
Other risk factors	Obesity, acute smoking cessation, and opioid use are also risk factors
High-risk profiles	Female, young age, and diminished physical health for age

---

Box 1
Types of surgery most prone to chronic postsurgical pain development

- Mastectomy
- Thoracotomy
- Open cholecystectomy
- Nephrectomy
- Sternotomy
- Knee arthroplasty
- Amputation
- Inguinal and pelvic surgeries

---

1. *Surgery type:* Certain types of surgery are more likely to produce CPSP. Those procedures are mastectomy, thoracotomy, open cholecystectomy, nephrectomy, sternotomy, total knee arthroplasty, amputation, inguinal, and pelvic surgeries.[16] Strategies to reduce risks associated with the type of surgical procedure include reducing surgical time and reducing the invasive nature of the procedure. As an example, laparoscopic alternatives have a lower incidence of chronic pain development than open procedures.

2. *Anesthetic type:* The goal of surgical anesthesia is to target the receptors within the nociceptive and neuropathic pathways to reduce surgical stress response. However, certain types of anesthesia can be counterproductive in the goal of reducing the risk of CPSP. General inhalation anesthesia appears to activate a key nociceptive ion channel and enhance nerve-mediated postoperative pain.[17] High-dose and high-potency opioids, particularly remifentanil, can produce opioid-induced hyperalgesia and increase the risk of CPSP as well. The use of regional and local anesthesia can reduce the incidence of CPSP by reducing the pain signals transmitted to the spinal cord, which reduces the likelihood of central sensitization.[18]

3. *Preoperative pain:* Proper pain management during the preoperative period may lead to a reduction in CPSP. Pain at the site of surgery or anywhere else on the body is a risk factor for CPSP and should be addressed. The use of preoperative anti-inflammatory agents, preoperative regional anesthesia, and other alternative methods to reduce preoperative pain have been shown to reduce the incidence of CPSP.[19]

4. *Mental health:* Several studies suggest that psychological/psychosocial preoperative patient factors directly impact the pathophysiological surgical stress response, which may elevate the risk of developing CPSP. Depression and anxiety may also interfere with wound healing, immune responses, inflammatory reduction, pain perception, and care plan compliance.[20] Therefore, depression and anxiety should be addressed prior to surgery.[21] There are a number of options that can be utilized prior to surgery to address these issues. They include cognitive-behavioral therapy including appropriate preoperative teaching, relaxation techniques, hypnosis, coping strategies, and pharmaceutical interventions.

5. *Other potential risk factors:* Obesity is one of the risk factors of CPSP that can be addressed. Inflammation and oxidative stress associated with obesity and diet are thought to be one of the pathophysiological causes of chronic pain.[22] There is an overall positive effect of weight loss on chronic pain, with no specific diet showing superiority over another. This suggests that whichever approach works best for the

individual patient may help in modulating pain physiology.[23] In addition, preoperative weight loss may have a positive impact on postsurgical recovery.

Smoking as a risk factor may be a difficult problem to address. It appears that attempting to stop smoking postsurgery contributes to the possible development of CPSP. A better strategy would appear to be cessation of smoking prior to surgery, which would benefit the patient in many ways including a possible reduction of CPSP in comparison to those who stopped smoking postoperatively.

Addressing the CPSP risk related to preoperative opioid use is another complicated issue. Long-term opioid use has a multitude of associated negative consequences, among them is the possible risks of CPSP. It appears that an effort to reduce opioid use prior to surgery, and the utilization of nonopioid treatments for postoperative pain, such as regional anesthesia, nonsteroidal anti-inflammatory drugs (NSAIDs), nonpharmaceutical modalities, and so forth, would be in the best interest of the patient and the most likely strategy to reduce the risk of CPSP associated with opioid use.

MEDICAL/PHARMACOLOGIC MANAGEMENT

Once the condition of CPSP is diagnosed, it can be extremely difficult to treat. For that reason, pre-emptive strategies are superior to postoperative diagnostic treatment. If preemptive strategies are either not utilized or ineffective in preventing CPSP, the rapid diagnosis of CPSP and aggressive treatment is the next best solution. The longer the condition is untreated, the more difficult it will become to find a solution.

Nonsteroidal Anti-inflammatory Drugs

NSAIDs work by preventing the enzyme cyclooxygenase from producing the proin-flammation hormone prostaglandin. Excess inflammation can contribute to CPSP. There are several drugs that target the production of cyclooxygenase. Two of the most common over-the-counter drugs are ibuprofen and naproxen, while the most common prescription drug is celecoxib. The use of NSAIDs preoperatively and post-operatively for even a short period of time (less than 24 hours) shows significant impact 12 months out on postoperative pain.[24]

Acetaminophen

Acetaminophen does not possess significant anti-inflammatory properties but instead addresses the production of prostaglandins in the central nervous system rather than at the site of injury like true NSAIDs. Acetaminophen is available over the counter and as a perioperative intravenous infusion. Studies do demonstrate that the use of intravenous acetaminophen in the perioperative period does reduce the incidence of persistent pain, although the mechanism of action is unknown.[25]

Opioids

Opioids have been the mainstay of acute postoperative pain treatment, but their long-term use has produced significant negative consequences in terms of addiction, progressive tolerance, hyperalgesia, and even death. It is clear that those who are treated with opioids for chronic pain have shown higher rates of substance abuse disorders. Escalating doses of opioids can result in increased sensitivity to noxious stimulation and create a condition known as "OIH".[26] However, opioids continue to be prescribed for long-term use in those with chronic pain because using alternative treatments can be resource intensive, hard to validate, ineffective, costly, and time consuming.

The use of opioids for CPSP is controversial. It appears that proper monitoring, a motivated patient, and a knowledgeable provider can effectively use opioids for

CPSP treatment while avoiding the most significant consequences of misuse.[27] The goal of any chronic pain treatment should be to reduce, not escalate, the use of opioids over time and find alternative treatments that can be effective for the individual patient.

Antidepressants

There are several antidepressants on the market today and most are part of 1 of 3 classifications: tricyclic antidepressants, selective serotonin reuptake inhibitors (SSRIs), and norepinephrine serotonin reuptake inhibitors.

Amitriptyline is a tricyclic antidepressant that has been used for the treatment of chronic pain. It has been used for many years as a first-line treatment of chronic pain and continues to show promise. The major issue with tricyclic antidepressants is the potential for serious side effects. However, they continue to be recommended as a treatment of neuropathic pain and CPSP.[28]

There are several SSRIs on the market and many of them have been studied for their effectiveness in the treatment of various types of chronic pain. It does appear that SSRIs do have a positive impact on most chronic pain conditions including CPSP.[29] SSRIs have a more favorable side effect profile than tricyclic antidepressants.

Serotonin norepinephrine reuptake inhibitors, like SSRIs, have a safer side effect profile than tricyclic antidepressants and appear to be equally effective in treating chronic pain. In addition to providing analgesic and some anti-inflammatory capabilities, their mood stabilizing capabilities also promote care plan compliance and better treatment outcomes.[30]

Anticonvulsants

Pregabalin and gabapentin are 2 anticonvulsants that have been used to treat neuropathic pain and central sensitization. They have been found to be effective for diabetic neuropathy, postherpetic neuralgia, and trigeminal neuralgia. Some studies suggest that these anticonvulsants may play a role in the treatment of central sensitization conditions like CPSP. The use of these medications for CPSP is most effective when taken in conjunction with other medications and not as a first-line or primary treatment.[31]

N-methyl-D-aspartate Inhibitors

NMDA receptors have been found to have a critical link in neurotransmission and perception. In chronic pain conditions like CPSP, these pathways become dysfunctional and hyperactive. Inhibiting or reducing NMDA receptor activity produces analgesic effects during chronic pain conditions.[32]

Ketamine has been used since the 1970s in anesthesia as a dissociative agent for sedation during minor diagnostic and surgical procedures. In high concentrations, its side effect profile became unacceptable, and the drug became less popular because of these side effects of hallucinations, nausea, hypertension, impaired coordination, and psychosis. However, ketamine has recently emerged as an effective treatment of posttraumatic stress syndrome (PTSD), neuropathic pain, depression, and chronic pain when used at much lower doses.[33] At these lower doses, the concerning side effects are rare, and the benefit in some patients appears to be significant.

The Office of Research and Development for Veterans Affairs reports some promise in the development of an NMDA inhibitor that can treat PTSD, depression, and chronic pain without the serious side effects of ketamine.[34]

Topical Anesthetics and Distracting Agents

Topical agents offer advantages over oral medications. They can often target the site of pain more effectively and bypass first-pass metabolism. They typically have a much lower systemic impact that reduces unwanted side effects on other organs especially the gastrointestinal system, kidneys, and liver. Studies suggest that topical agents offer an effective alternative to systemic therapies in the treatment of chronic and neuropathic pain.[35]

Topical agents have the same mechanism of action as their oral counterparts. They include NSAIDs, local anesthetics, and distraction agents like capsaicin. Distraction agents work to reduce the function of nociceptors in the skin by creating a local hypersensitivity reaction. The depolarization of local nociceptors reduces pain signals to the brain. They have no impact on the treatment of the inflammatory process and so they do not serve as a direct treatment of the causation of CPSP.

EMERGING THERAPIES/EMERGING TREATMENT

Some therapies for CPSP that need more research to determine effectiveness are hypnosis, acupuncture, cannabinoids, and cryotherapy. These alternative therapies have a place for individualized treatment but appear to be more effective when combined with conventional treatment.

When a specific nerve or group of nerves can be identified as the causative of CPSP, and they have no motor activity, cryoablation, radiofrequency ablation, or surgical intervention may provide a solution (**Table 4**).

CHALLENGES

The challenge of CPSP is finding the right treatment. Chronic pain, especially CPSP, is often ignored because it is an unexpected result of a corrective surgical procedure. The longer the problem is undiagnosed, the more difficult it is to treat.

Even when treatment is initiated, compliance with alternative therapies can be challenging as well. Opioids are the most frequently prescribed treatment of pain, but the

Table 4
Effectiveness of treatments of chronic postsurgical pain

Treatment	Effectiveness
Nursing intervention	Compassion and empathy reduce CPSP risk
NSAIDs	Significant benefit when used presurgery or postsurgery for even <24 h
Acetaminophen	Perioperative use reduces incidence of CPSP
Opioids	Long-term use is discouraged
Antidepressants	Some analgesic impact along with mood stabilization and care plan compliance
Anticonvulsants	Most beneficial when used in conjunction with other treatments
NMDA inhibitors	Low-dose use appears to provide value in the treatment of chronic pain
Topical agents	Topical NSAIDs, anesthetic agents, and distractors show treatment value
Other therapies	Hypnosis, acupuncture, cannabinoids, ablation, and surgery show promise

difficulty in proper utilization of opioids for chronic pain has made them a poor long-term strategy.

It is important that any treatment strategy includes the patient, the family, support systems, other providers, and an individualized treatment plan. Without compliance from everyone involved, success is unlikely.

SUMMARY

CPSP is a very common complication from surgery. Diagnosis of CPSP can be difficult and treatment can be complex. The condition often hinders surgical recovery and can create patient dissatisfaction. It is important that any preoperative evaluation include a risk analysis for CPSP and that mitigation strategies be identified that may reduce the risk of CPSP development.

Prevention and treatment of CPSP is the responsibility of the entire health care team. Nursing intervention is critical. Anesthesia care tailored to those at high risk is essential to prevention. Surgeon awareness of the risk can help to incorporate mitigation strategies into the surgical plan. The goal should be prevention, but if CPSP develops in a postsurgical patient, it is important that CPSP be identified as quickly as possible and aggressive treatment be implemented. The longer the condition persists, the more difficult it is to treat.

As with any chronic pain condition, the goal should be improvement in activities of daily living. It is often unrealistic to promise complete pain relief. Setting realistic goals is essential to success and return to homeostasis.

CLINICS CARE POINTS

- CPSP is a common complication of surgery.
- Risk factors for CPSP should be part of any preoperative evaluation.
- When risk factors are identified, mitigation strategies should be attempted.
- Nursing intervention is critical.
- Tailored anesthesia care is essential.
- Surgery mitigation strategies are possible.
- Treatment should begin as soon as possible and include a multimodal approach.
- Avoidance of long-term opioid use should be a goal.

DISCLOSURE

The author has no commercial or financial conflicts to disclose related to this article.

REFERENCES

1. Rikard SM, Strahan AE, Schmit KM, et al. Chronic pain among adults - United States, 2019-2021. MMWR Morb Mortal Wkly Rep 2023;72(15):379–85.
2. Treede RD, Rief W, Barke A, et al. A classification of chronic pain for ICD-11. Pain 2015;156(6):1003–7.
3. Haroutiunian S, Nikolajsen L, Finnerup NB, et al. The neuropathic component in persistent postsurgical pain: a systematic literature review. Pain 2013;154(1): 95–102.

4. Jensen MP, Chodroff MJ, Dworkin RH. The impact of neuropathic pain on health-related quality of life: review and implications. Neurology 2007;68(15):1178–82.

5. Emerson AJ, Oxendine RH, Chandler LE, et al. Patient and provider Attitudes, Beliefs, and biases that contribute to a marginalized process of care and outcomes in chronic Musculoskeletal pain: a systematic review-Part I: clinical care. Pain Med 2022;23(4):655–68.

6. Courtenay M, Carey N. The impact and effectiveness of nurse-led care in the management of acute and chronic pain: a review of the literature. J Clin Nurs 2008;17(15):2001–13.

7. Leknes S, Bastian B. The benefits of pain. Review of Philosophy and Psychology 2014;5(1):57–70.

8. Yam MF, Loh YC, Tan CS, et al. General pathways of pain sensation and the major Neurotransmitters involved in pain Regulation. Int J Mol Sci 2018;19(8). https://doi.org/10.3390/ijms19082164.

9. Feizerfan A, Sheh G. Transition from acute to chronic pain. Cont Educ Anaesth Crit Care Pain 2014;15(2):98–102.

10. Bruce J, Quinlan J. Chronic post surgical pain. Reviews in Pain 2011;5(3):23–9.

11. Schug SA, Lavand'homme P, Barke A, et al. The IASP classification of chronic pain for ICD-11: chronic postsurgical or posttraumatic pain. Pain 2019;160(1).

12. Montes A, Roca G, Cantillo J, et al. Presurgical risk model for chronic postsurgical pain based on 6 clinical predictors: a prospective external validation. Pain 2020;161(11):2611–8.

13. Liu XM, Zhao Y, Zhang LY, et al. Effects of preoperative current smoking on chronic postsurgical pain in thoracic surgery: a retrospective cohort study. Am J Transl Res 2023;15(3):2256–67.

14. Lee M, Silverman SM, Hansen H, et al. A comprehensive review of opioid-induced hyperalgesia. Pain Physician 2011;14(2):145–61.

15. Fukazawa K, Rodriguez PJ, Fong CT, et al. Perioperative opioid Use and chronic post-surgical pain after Liver Transplantation: a Single center Observational study. Journal of Cardiothoracic and Vascular Anesthesia 2020;34(7):1815–21.

16. Correll D. Chronic postoperative pain: recent findings in understanding and management. F1000Res 2017;6:1054.

17. Matta JA, Cornett PM, Miyares RL, et al. General anesthetics activate a nociceptive ion channel to enhance pain and inflammation. Proc Natl Acad Sci U S A 2008;105(25):8784–9.

18. Rivat C, Bollag L, Richebé P. Mechanisms of regional anaesthesia protection against hyperalgesia and pain chronicization. Curr Opin Anaesthesiol 2013;26(5):621–5.

19. Gerbershagen HJ, Ozgür E, Dagtekin O, et al. Preoperative pain as a risk factor for chronic post-surgical pain - six month follow-up after radical prostatectomy. Eur J Pain 2009;13(10):1054–61.

20. Villa G, Lanini I, Amass T, et al. Effects of psychological interventions on anxiety and pain in patients undergoing major elective abdominal surgery: a systematic review. Perioperat Med 2020;9(1):38.

21. Giusti EM, Lacerenza M, Manzoni GM, et al. Psychological and psychosocial predictors of chronic postsurgical pain: a systematic review and meta-analysis. Pain 2021;162(1):10–30.

22. Kaushik AS, Strath LJ, Sorge RE. Dietary interventions for treatment of chronic pain: oxidative stress and inflammation. Pain and Therapy 2020;9(2):487–98.

23. Field R, Pourkazemi F, Turton J, et al. Dietary interventions are Beneficial for patients with chronic pain: a systematic review with meta-analysis. Pain Med 2020; 22(3):694–714.

24. van Helmond N, Steegers MA, Filippini-de Moor GP, et al. Hyperalgesia and persistent pain after Breast Cancer surgery: a prospective Randomized Controlled trial with Perioperative COX-2 inhibition. PLoS One 2016;11(12): e0166601.

25. Koyuncu O, Hakimoglu S, Ugur M, et al. Acetaminophen reduces acute and persistent incisional pain after hysterectomy. Ann Ital Chir 2018;89:357–66.

26. Angst MS, Clark JD. Opioid-induced hyperalgesia: a qualitative systematic review. Anesthesiology 2006;104(3):570–87.

27. Nadeau SE, Wu JK, Lawhern RA. Opioids and chronic pain: an Analytic review of the clinical Evidence. Front Pain Res (Lausanne) 2021;2:721357.

28. Moore RA, Derry S, Aldington D, et al. Amitriptyline for neuropathic pain in adults. Cochrane Database Syst Rev 2015;2015(7):Cd008242.

29. Patetsos E, Horjales-Araujo E. Treating chronic pain with SSRIs: what do We Know? Pain Res Manag 2016;2016:2020915.

30. Robinson C, Dalal S, Chitneni A, et al. A look at commonly utilized serotonin Noradrenaline reuptake inhibitors (SNRIs) in chronic pain. Health Psychol Res 2022;10(3):32309.

31. Wiffen PJ, Derry S, Bell RF, et al. Gabapentin for chronic neuropathic pain in adults. Cochrane Database Syst Rev 2017;6(6):Cd007938.

32. Li XH, Miao HH, Zhuo M. NMDA receptor Dependent long-term Potentiation in chronic pain. Neurochem Res 2019;44(3):531–8.

33. Voute M, Riant T, Amodéo J-M, et al. Ketamine in chronic pain: a Delphi survey. Eur J Pain 2022;26(4):873–87.

34. Richman M. Drug that acts like ketamine but without the potential for abuse or psychotic effects. Available at: https://www.research.va.gov/currents/1217-Cognitive-drug-yields-positive-lab-results.cfm. [Accessed 14 January 2024].

35. Stanos SP, Galluzzi KE. Topical therapies in the management of chronic pain. PGM (Postgrad Med) 2013;125(sup1):25–33.

36. Rosenberger DC, Pogatzki-Zahn EM. Chronic post-surgical pain - update on incidence, risk factors and preventive treatment options. BJA Educ 2022;22(5): 190–6.

Optimizing Patient Comfort
Palliative Pain Management for Nurses in Critical Care Settings

Ami Bhatt, PhD, DNP, MBA, RN[a],*, Avani Bhatt, MSN, RN[b],
Debra Sullivan, PhD, MSN, RN, CNE[a]

KEYWORDS

- Palliative care • SDOH • Nurse perceptions • Assessment for palliative care
- Intensive care unit, ICU • Patient-centered care • End-of-life care
- Family-centered care

KEY POINTS

- Palliative care focuses primarily on comfort measures throughout a serious illness while emphasizing quality of life rather than prolonging life.
- A holistic and comprehensive assessment is essential for effective pain management, incorporating both pharmacologic and nonpharmacologic approaches.
- Critical care nurses often face barriers due to lack of training in palliative care, high-intensity environments, and care coordination.

INTRODUCTION

Palliative care focuses on the relief from the symptoms and stress of chronic or acute illness when the patient or family seeks comfort measures. End-of-life care is often influenced by evolving medical practices and religious organizations. The concept of palliative care focuses primarily on comfort measures while emphasizing quality of life rather than prolonging life. Since establishing the first palliative care program in a hospital setting in the 1980s, there has been a growing recognition of the need for patient-centered comfort care.[1] Comfort care can take place in any health care setting. Recent efforts have focused on improving access to palliative care and addressing gaps in its application, including developing predictive tools and algorithms to identify patients who would benefit from early palliative care interventions. The World Health Organization defines palliative care as improving the quality of life

[a] College of Nursing, Walden University, 100 South Washington Avenue, Suite 900, Minneapolis, MN 55401, USA; [b] Trinity Health-Ann Arbor Hospital, 5301 McAuley Drive, Ypsilanti, MI 48197, USA
* Corresponding author.
E-mail address: ami.bhatt@mail.waldenu.edu

Crit Care Nurs Clin N Am 36 (2024) 597–608
https://doi.org/10.1016/j.cnc.2024.07.003 ccnursing.theclinics.com
0899-5885/24/© 2024 Elsevier Inc. All rights reserved, including for text and data mining, AI training, and similar technologies.

for patients and families dealing with life-threatening illnesses, irrespective of prognosis.[2] This perspective challenges the misconception that palliative care is synonymous with end-of-life care, highlighting its applicability throughout serious illness.

The critical care environment often involves complex technologies and sensory overload and is designed to prevent morbidity and mortality. Creating conditions that can reduce suffering was the key priority of hospice and palliative care.[3] The high mortality rate in intensive care units (ICUs) underscores the need for effective palliative care interventions, which can alleviate suffering and enhance the quality of life even amidst aggressive treatments. Critical care nurses spend considerable time with patients and families and are uniquely positioned to integrate palliative care principles into their practice. Still, they often face barriers due to a lack of comprehensive training and understanding of palliative care concepts.

BACKGROUND

Throughout history, religious organizations have administered care for the dying.[1] Cicely Saunders was a British nurse, and social worker recognized as having formed the tenets of the first modern hospice.[1,3] Dr. Saunders presented a lecture in the United States in 1963 detailing holistic care with aggressive symptom control at end-of-life care.[1] Elisabeth Kubler-Ross brought further attention to the issue, believing that terminal patients progress through 5 stages of the end-of-life journey.[1] A Canadian doctor, Balfour Mound, is credited for the term "palliative care" in 1974, describing a treatment for symptom relief.[1,4] The first hospital-based palliative care program came to the United States in the late 1980s.[1] Palliative care is now a board-certified specialty for nurses and advanced practice nurses through the Hospice and Palliative Credentialing Center.[5]

The critical care environment today is complicated and daunting to a patient suffering a serious illness due to foreign machines and sensory overload.[6] The goal of intensive care in this environment is to decrease mortality and prevent morbidity.[7] Despite advancements in technology, the mortality rate in the ICU remains high, with 1 in 5 patients not surviving.[8] Critical care nurses spend more time with patients and families, can lower distress, and offer comfort measures such as palliative care and curative therapies.[9] Nurses are the most common health care providers working in interdisciplinary palliative care teams; therefore, it is essential that they can offer patients information on palliative care.[9,10] During the last decade, knowledge about palliative care has increased, but studies show a lack of understanding of how to interpret and apply palliative care concepts.[11,12]

According to the World Health Organization, palliative care aims to improve the quality of life for patients and their families when facing life-threatening illnesses, whether physical, psychological, social, or spiritual.[2] Historically, palliative care was focused on alleviating suffering at end-of-life, but now it is a best practice for patients facing a life-threatening health condition.[13] The common perception is that palliative care is the same as end-of-life care. Still, specialized palliative care can be provided with life-prolonging treatment, contributing to better symptom management and quality of life with less physical discomfort.[14] The American Association of Critical Care Nurses differentiates palliative care from end-of-life care, primarily because palliative care is appropriate at any time in the trajectory of a serious illness and does not replace curative intervention where end-of-life is associated with Hospice organizations providing patient care before death.[15]

A consensus-based definition of palliative care was developed by more than 450 palliative care workers from around the world.[13] This new definition purports that palliative care should be implemented based on need rather than prognosis and applies to all care settings.[13] The new definition is found below:

PC is the active holistic care of individuals across all ages with SHS (suffering is health related when it is associated with illness or injury of any kind. Health-related suffering is serious when it cannot be relieved without medical intervention and when it compromises physical, social, spiritual, and/or emotional functioning. Retrieved from http://pallipedia. org/serious-health-related-suffering-shs/) because of severe illness (severe illness is a condition that carries a high risk of mortality, negatively impacts quality of life and daily function, and/or is burdensome in symptoms, treatments, or caregiver stress. Available from http://pallipedia.org/serious-illness/) and especially of those near the end of life. It aims to improve the quality of life of patients, their families, and their caregivers.

PC

- Includes, prevention, early identification, comprehensive assessment, and management of physical issues, including pain and other distressing symptoms, psychological distress, spiritual distress, and social needs. Whenever possible, these interventions must be evidence based.
- Provides support to help patients live as fully as possible until death by facilitating effective communication, helping them, and their families determine goals of care.
- Is applicable throughout the course of an illness, according to the patient's needs is provided in conjunction with disease-modifying therapies whenever needed.
- May positively influence the course of illness. Intends neither to hasten nor to postpone death, affirms life, and recognizes dying as a natural process.
- Provides support to the family and caregivers during the patients' illness, and in their own bereavement.
- Is delivered recognizing and respecting the cultural values and beliefs of the patient and family.
- Is applicable throughout all health care settings (place of residence and institutions) and in all levels (primary to tertiary).
- Can be provided by professionals with basic PC training.
- Requires specialist PC with a multiprofessional team for referral of complex cases.

To achieve PC integration, governments should.

- Adopt adequate policies and norms that include PC in health laws, national health programs, and national health budgets.
- Ensure that insurance plans integrate PC as a component of programs.
- Ensure access to essential medicines and technologies for pain relief and PC, including pediatric formulations.
- Ensure that PC is part of all health services (from community health-based programs to hospitals), that everyone is assessed, and that all staff can provide basic PC with specialist teams available for referral and consultation.
- Ensure access to adequate PC for vulnerable groups, including children and older persons.
- Engage with universities, academia, and teaching hospitals to include PC research and PC training as an integral component of ongoing education, including basic, intermediate, specialist, and continuing education.
  PC $1/4$ palliative care; SHS $1/4$ serious health-related suffering.[13]

Access to palliative care has been on the rise in the United States. Despite this, only half of all patients who need palliative care actually receive it.[16] 1 problem is a shortage of palliative care providers and the overuse of aggressive care.[17] Several prognostic tools in palliative care aim to identify terminally ill patients early enough to plan for end-of-life care, but these are time-consuming chart reviews.[18] Unfortunately, in the ICU setting, the prognosis is often unclear, necessitating the need for early initiation of palliative care interventions.[19] In a recent study to address this problem, a deep neural network was developed using an algorithm to interface with the electronic health records each night to identify patients with a positive prediction of who would benefit from palliative care, allowing the palliative care team to be proactive in reaching out to patients.[17]

Decision-making, aligning treatment with the patient's goals, providing emotional support for families, and managing symptoms are fundamental elements of palliative care and should be standard practices in critical care.[19] However, when life-sustaining therapies are no longer effective, patients may be unable to make decisions. Advanced directives should guide decisions, but the health care team often makes decisions.[7] Critical care nurses will need to have appropriate discussions with the patient's family to help them accept a bad prognosis and the need for limiting life support.[20] In a 2023 study of ICU nurses, it was found that nurses understand the anxiety of relatives. Still, there is a need for further staff training related to cultural diversity, including patients' and their relatives' religious and spiritual values and beliefs in palliative and end-of-life care.[20]

Palliative care in the ICU has emerged as a core component of ICU care.[19] Basic palliative care can be provided by any health care professional and includes symptom management and discussions about advanced care planning. A multidisciplinary team offers professional palliative care with advanced training based on different palliative care models.[19]

Nursing Education and Training

Typical training for a registered nurse offers the necessary skills to care for dying patients, but a specialist in palliative care, either a registered nurse or an advanced practice nurse, has expert knowledge in pathophysiology, advanced pain and symptom assessment skills, communication, and care planning.[9] In 2017, the American Nurses Association and the Hospice and Palliative Nurses Association (HPNA) recommended the adoption of End of Life Nursing Education Consortium (ELNEC) curricula as the standard for palliative care education.[9] HPNA offers various certifications in hospice and palliative care for nurses.[5] Since 2000, the American Association of Colleges of Nursing, ELNEC, and the City of Hope have collaborated to provide nursing faculty, staff development educators, and specialty nurses with training in palliative care so that they can teach the components of ELNEC to nurses and nursing students.[21] The curriculum focuses on core end-of-life and palliative care areas and specialized modules, including one for the critical care nurse.[21]

In summary, historically, palliative care was focused on alleviating suffering at end-of-life, but now it is a best practice for patients facing a life-threatening health condition.[13] Palliative care is a core component of ICU care and can be provided as basic or advanced palliative care. There is specialized training for critical care nurses who want more education on palliative care through ELNEC[21] or to become certified in palliative care through HPNA.[5] Critical care nurses need to understand the components of palliative care to provide patients with holistic care to alleviate physical and emotional symptoms while communicating appropriately with family.

PAIN MANAGEMENT APPROACHES

Pain management involves a holistic assessment to determine the best approach to pain management. It involves physical, psychological, social determinates of health (SDOH), and spiritual assessment. Specialized palliative pain management includes both pharmaceutical and non-pharmaceutical patient and family-centered approaches.

Assessment of Social Determinates of Health and Other Essential Factors

A critical care nurse must conduct a thorough assessment to manage pain effectively in the ICU. Various barriers within the health care system prevent adequate acknowledgment of patient pain perception. These barriers include a lack of nursing knowledge regarding pain assessment and management, missed communication between the interdisciplinary team regarding pain levels, and an absence of standardized guidelines for pain control.[22] To care for the critical patient, the nurse should perform a well-rounded pain assessment by including patient behaviors and their relation to pain levels.[22] Using subjective and objective information, the nurse can communicate the pain level to providers and develop a plan for analgesics and non-pharmacologic approaches to reduce pain.[22]

In addition to using nonverbal and verbal cues, the nurse should take a step further and address the SDOH related to patient care. Addressing potential barriers to care, including race, gender, disability, age, religion, and health literacy, is key to performing holistic care.[23] While addressing pain in the critical care setting, the interdisciplinary team should consider all factors hindering the reporting and treatment of pain. Research has shown that higher levels of implicit bias within health care workers regarding race directly led to lower quality of care for minorities.[24] Reviewing the key factors of the acute critical care situation and social determinants of health will contribute to holistic care.

Furthermore, reviewing health literacy with the patient and family will help to construct heightened and more meaningful care and education.[23] In any health care setting, patient education and care plans should be laid out in a way that is clear for the patient. Addressing palliative medicine in a critical situation can cause an uproar of emotion, especially if explained poorly. Palliative care improves the quality of life of patients and families dealing with life-threatening illnesses by enhancing comfort levels and providing holistic care.[2] Differentiating between hospice and palliative care is also key, ensuring the care team provides clear guidelines for end goals.

Another imperative topic to discuss between pain and social determinants of health is the current substance use disorder crisis within the United States. Due to the heightened abuse of common analgesics, unnecessarily restrictive regulations on these medications directly reduce access to palliative medicine.[2] With strict regulations on analgesic medications, it becomes difficult to maintain comfort in both palliative and end-of-life care. Adequately assessing pain in the critical care patient involves addressing signs and symptoms while considering outside factors.

Perceptions: Influences on Beliefs, Stereotypes, and Biases

When discussing palliative medicine, it is critical to consider the religious and spiritual implications for the patients and families. Often, a patient's decision-making in palliative care situations is influenced by religious and spiritual beliefs and a sense of meaning in life as.[25] To approach a serious illness or end of life, many patients and families rely on the physical, social, psychological, and spiritual dimensions of life.[25] Considering all of these aspects allows the health care team to provide holistic care meaningfully. Spirituality at the end of life helps patients make sense of their lives and enhances feelings of autonomy in decision-making.[25] Reviewing the spiritual needs of critically ill patients can help guide decision-making skills and enhance the overall comfort that the patient and family feel.

In addition to spirituality, palliative medicine may be perceived differently based on religious views. The discussion of various religious and cultural beliefs regarding palliative care begins with the thoughts about pain as a whole. For example, Christianity emphasizes comfort for the patient as long as side effects are minimal from analgesic use.[26] Similarly, Judaism focuses on pain medication for comfort. However, there are concerns about the decreased level of consciousness and the impact of sedation from pain medication.[25] Buddhism, however, focuses on the mental well-being of the patient and requests health care professionals to focus on the mental health of the client to distract from any physical suffering.[25] With knowledge of the patient's religious beliefs and values, the nurse and health care team can cater palliative care in accordance with these beliefs. While analgesics are one solution to pain management in the critical care setting, some patients may value a nonpharmacologic approach to pain management.

Pain is subjective. Therefore, stereotypical ideas surround this area of patient care. Studies have shown that while women are at a higher likelihood of having chronic pain, pain medication is prescribed less to women when compared to men.[27] In fact, chronic pain is stigmatized among the female patient population, which leads to improper conclusions on psychological reasons for pain rather than somatic.[27] 1 solution to help the stereotypes surrounding pain is to promote pain education and enhance pain assessment knowledge among health care workers.[27] Reducing stereotypical thoughts and behaviors can help enhance just care for patients in the critical care setting experiencing pain.

While most of the pain and palliative medicine considerations arise from patients' thoughts and beliefs, implicit bias among health care workers is equally important to discuss. Implicit bias can be explained as unknown stereotypical thoughts that have an impact on the patient-physician relationship.[24] 1 study depicts the impact implicit bias can have, as physicians with higher levels of implicit bias provided lower quality care to Black patients, including less prescriptions for opioids and reduced patient-centered care pain communication and assessments.[23] A holistic pain assessment requires well-rounded knowledge of the patient and diminished implicit bias among health care workers.

Pharmacologic Approaches to Palliative Pain Management

One of the first-line methods for treating pain in the ICU setting is pharmacologic approaches, particularly with analgesics and opioids. Pharmacologic pain management includes nonsteroidal anti-inflammatory drugs (NSAIDs) and opioid analgesics.[28] In fact, opioid analgesics are the gold standard for pain management in palliative care and at the end of life, as they provide the most pain relief.[28]

Pharmacologic interventions are integral to managing symptoms that cannot be adequately addressed non-pharmacologically. These interventions aim to control pain, alleviate distressing symptoms, and enhance comfort. Some of these interventions include analgesics, including opioids and NSAIDs; adjuvant medications that may include corticosteroids, anticonvulsants, and antidepressants; sedatives and anxiolytics; antiemetics; and, finally, palliative care for non-pain symptoms, such as antibiotics and diuretics.[7]

There are a multitude of suggestions for managing patients in the ICU. With 2 main models, the integrative and consultative models, palliative care principles and interventions can be applied more readily. In the integrative model, palliative care interventions and principles are embedded into daily practice by the ICU team; with the consultative model, there is a focus on the involvement of palliative care consultants in the care of ICU patients, which may include social workers, spiritual care personnel, and nurse practitioners. Using these models would allow the application of measures to address the social, psychological, and spiritual domains.[7] While pharmacologic methods are essential for managing acute symptoms and providing relief, nonpharmacologic strategies can enhance overall comfort, address emotional and psychological needs, and support patients and families through the complexities of serious illness.

Ultimately, personalized care that combines these approaches and is tailored to the patient's specific needs and preferences is crucial for achieving the best possible outcomes in palliative care. This holistic approach improves symptom management and contributes to a more compassionate, interdisciplinary, and supportive care experience.

Nonpharmacologic Approaches to Palliative Pain Management

Nonpharmacologic methods for treating palliative pain go above medication administration. Simple interventions such as repositioning, proper hygiene care, and extra cushioning to prevent pressure ulcers can enhance comfort for these patients.[28] Furthermore, counseling and organizing palliative care or if appropriate end-of-life goals can help increase feelings of autonomy while alleviating anxiety.[28]

Nonpharmacologic interventions are essential components of a holistic approach to palliative care. They focus on improving patient comfort and well-being without the use of medications. These strategies can complement pharmacologic treatments and often address the broader aspects of patient care, including physical, psychological, and emotional needs. Multiple strategies can be used to implement nonpharmacologic approaches, and some of them include:

Repositioning for comfort includes frequent repositioning; creating a calm environment; psychological support and counseling as needed; complementary therapies, such as music therapy, aromatherapy, or massage therapy; and education, communication, and collaboration. Clear but compassionate communication is necessary to empower patients to make informed decisions.

Palliative Pain Assessment Tools

Critical care nurses can utilize foundational pain assessment tools. Regarding pain assessment in critically ill patients, the Behavioral Pain Scale and Critical Care Pain Observation Tool are used for mechanically ventilated patients.[29] Since these patients are unable to state a pain level subjectively, behaviors are measured to evaluate pain.[29] For those patients able to express pain levels, the tools listed in the table are feasible.

Holistic Approach and Future Directions

To approach palliative care holistically, the critical nurse must consider the patient as a whole being. A person and family-centered holistic approach addresses physical, psychological, social, and spiritual suffering.[2] Assessing the patient using adequate tools and addressing alternative factors will help formulate the most appropriate care plan. Considering the religious and spiritual beliefs and the social determinants of health impacting the patient and family will help proceed with palliative measures and overall enhanced comfort.[23] Furthermore, ensuring collaboration between nurses and physicians for an adequate analgesic plan will help control pain levels.[22] Optimizing patient comfort requires a holistic assessment and consideration of various outside factors to formulate a well-rounded plan for enhanced comfort.

BARRIERS

Palliative care delivery in the ICU encounters numerous challenges that significantly impact its effectiveness. Cultural and attitudinal barriers among ICU health care providers often equate palliative care with end-of-life measures or relinquishing curative treatments. This barrier leads to hesitancy in initiating discussions or referrals for palliative care services. In the ICU, characterized by high-stress environments and time constraints, communication frequently obstructs clear dialogue among health care teams, patients, and families regarding palliative care options, treatment preferences, and care goals. Prognostic uncertainty adds another layer of complexity, making it challenging to identify the optimal timing for introducing palliative care discussions or transitioning from aggressive treatments to comfort-focused care. Additionally, resource limitations may mean that ICUs need more dedicated palliative care teams or specialists, placing additional burdens on already stretched ICU staff who may lack specialized training in palliative care. Ethical dilemmas arise from balancing aggressive medical interventions with palliative care approaches, particularly when patients and families hold divergent expectations.

Moreover, varied family dynamics and decision-making processes can complicate care plans and discussions around palliative care. Inconsistent integration of palliative care principles into ICU protocols and documentation practices further contributes to variations in care quality. Regulatory and policy frameworks may not uniformly prioritize or support the provision of palliative care within ICUs, impacting its availability and accessibility. Addressing these barriers necessitates a comprehensive approach that includes educating health care providers, enhancing communication strategies, integrating palliative care seamlessly into ICU workflows, and fostering an institutional culture that prioritizes patient-centered care across the spectrum of illness.[23] An open and active dialogue between interdisciplinary team members can assist in eliminating many of the barriers.

OVERCOMING BARRIERS IN PALLIATIVE CARE

Effective communication and collaboration are foundational to providing high-quality palliative care. These measures ensure that patient care is coordinated, goals are aligned, and both patients and families are supported throughout the care process. These elements are crucial for managing complex cases, particularly in palliative settings, since addressing medical and emotional needs is essential. In a complex and evolving health care atmosphere, communication can provide many benefits to promote improved quality and safety. All aspects of care are addressed through open and honest discussions, clear and compassionate dialogue, and collaboration with the team. Coordination of care and team members working toward the same goals is also crucial.

CASE STUDY

Mr. John Doe is a 72-year-old male with Advanced Stage IV Lung Cancer with metastasis to the liver and bones. He has been admitted to the ICU with severe respiratory distress and acute exacerbation of chronic obstructive pulmonary disease. Currently, he is intubated and mechanically ventilated in the ICU and unresponsive to aggressive treatments.

Mr. John Doe was admitted to the ICU following a sudden deterioration in his respiratory function. Despite maximal medical interventions, his condition continued to decline. Given the advanced stage of his cancer and poor prognosis, the ICU team, along with the

Box 1
Case Study

Mr. D is a 72-year-old male with Advanced Stage IV Lung Cancer with metastasis to the liver and bones. He has been admitted to the ICU with severe respiratory distress and acute exacerbation of chronic obstructive pulmonary disease (COPD). Currently, he is intubated and mechanically ventilated in the ICU and unresponsive to aggressive treatments. Mr. D was admitted to the ICU following a sudden deterioration in his respiratory function. Despite maximal medical interventions, his condition continued to decline. Given the advanced stage of his cancer and poor prognosis, the ICU team, along with the palliative care team, discussed shifting the focus from curative to palliative care with his family. **Box 1** outlines the palliative care goals, care plan, and conclusions.

Palliative Care Plan for Mr. D:
1. Symptom Management:
   - Pain Management:
     - Initiate a continuous infusion of morphine for pain control.
     - Adjust doses based on pain assessment using non-verbal cues (eg, grimacing, restlessness).
   - Dyspnea Management:
     - Titrate sedatives (midazolam) to ease the sensation of breathlessness.
     - Optimize ventilator settings for comfort.
   - Anxiety Management:
     - Administer low-dose benzodiazepines for anxiety relief.
     - Provide a calm and quiet environment.
2. Emotional and Psychological Support:
   - Family Meetings:
     - Regularly schedule meetings with Mr. D's family to discuss his condition, prognosis, and care preferences.
     - Offer counseling services for family members.
   - Psychological Support:
     - Engage a clinical psychologist for emotional support.
     - Provide information on coping strategies and grief counseling.
3. Ethical and Spiritual Support:
   - Ethical Considerations:
     - Discuss and document advance directives.
     - Ensure that the care plan aligns with Mr. D's and his family's values and preferences.
   - Spiritual Care:
     - Facilitate visits from the hospital chaplain.
     - Support the family in performing any religious or cultural rituals.
4. Communication and Decision Making:
   - Family Conferences:
     - Hold regular interdisciplinary meetings involving the ICU team, palliative care team, and family.
     - Clearly communicate the shift from curative to comfort-focused care.
   - Advance Care Planning:
     - Discuss and implement DNR orders.
     - Plan for potential withdrawal of mechanical ventilation if agreed upon by the family.

Outcomes:
- Comfort: Mr. D's pain and dyspnea were effectively managed, ensuring he remained comfortable.
- Family Satisfaction: The family felt supported and well-informed throughout the process, appreciating the compassionate care provided.
- Ethical Resolution: The transition to palliative care respected Mr. D's wishes, ensuring a dignified end-of-life experience.

Reflections:
- Challenges:
  - Managing the complex symptoms of advanced cancer in an ICU setting.
  - Navigating emotional and ethical dilemmas with the family.

- Successes:
  - Effective symptom control and improved patient comfort.
  - Interdisciplinary collaboration ensures comprehensive care.
  - Enhanced family satisfaction and support during this difficult time.

Conclusion

This case highlights the importance of integrating palliative care into managing critically ill patients in the ICU. By addressing physical, emotional, and spiritual needs, palliative care ensures that patients like Mr. D receive holistic and compassionate care, ultimately improving their quality of life even in their final days.

palliative care team, discussed shifting the focus from curative to palliative care with his family. **Box 1** outlines the palliative care goals, care plan, and conclusions.

SUMMARY

In conclusion, the evolution of palliative care from its religious and historical roots to its current standing as a specialized medical discipline underscores its crucial role in enhancing the quality of life for patients with serious illnesses. The pioneering work of early figures such as Cicely Saunders and Elisabeth Kübler-Ross has laid a foundation that continues to guide modern practices, emphasizing the importance of symptom management, emotional support, and holistic care. The establishment of palliative care as a board-certified specialty reflects a significant advancement in addressing the complex needs of patients and their families, particularly in high-intensity settings such as the ICU.

Despite these advancements, challenges do remain. The critical care environment's inherent complexity can complicate the integration of palliative care, and barriers such as limited provider availability and misconceptions about the role of palliative care persist. Efforts to improve access through predictive tools and enhanced training for critical care nurses are steps in the right direction. Yet, a broader understanding and application of palliative care principles are essential.

As health care evolves, it is imperative to recognize that palliative care is not confined to end-of-life scenarios but is a fundamental aspect of managing severe illness at any stage. Ensuring that health care professionals are well-trained in palliative care, addressing the barriers to its implementation, and fostering a culture that values curative and comfort-oriented interventions will be vital to providing compassionate, patient-centered care. By bridging gaps in knowledge and practice, we can enhance the overall well-being of patients and their families, aligning medical care with the values and needs of those served.

CLINICS CARE POINTS

- Palliative care prioritizes comfort measures during serious illness, emphasizing the quality of life rather than extending it.
- Palliative care in the ICU has emerged as a core component of ICU care.
- Critical care nurses must holistically assess patients for appropriate pain management. Still, there is a need for further training related to cultural diversity, attitudinal biases, and communication with the health care team.
- It is crucial to ensure health care professionals are well-trained in palliative care, to address the barriers to its implementation, and to foster a culture that values both curative and comfort-oriented approaches.

DISCLOSURE

The authors have no commercial or financial conflicts to disclose.

REFERENCES

1. Lutz S. The history of hospice and palliative care. Curr Probl Cancer 2011;35(6): 304–9. https://doi.org/10.1016/j.currproblcancer.2011.10.004.
2. Palliative care. Available at: https://www.who.int/news-room/fact-sheets/detail/palliative-care. Accessed June 21, 2024.
3. Džakula A, Lončarek K, Vočanec D. Palliative care - too complex to make it simple. Croat Med J 2024;65(2):165–6.
4. Balfour Mount. Palliative care McGill. Available at: https://www.mcgill.ca/palliativecare/about-us/portraits/balfour-mount. Accessed June 21, 2024.
5. Certification. Adv expert care. Available at: https://www.advancingexpertcare.org/hpcc/. Accessed June 21, 2024.
6. Impact of critical care environment on patients | PDF | patient | nursing. Available at: https://www.scribd.com/document/626363488/impact-of-critical-care-environment-on-patients. Accessed June 21, 2024.
7. Mercadante S, Gregoretti C, Cortegiani A. Palliative care in intensive care units: why, where, what, who, when, how. BMC Anesthesiol 2018;18(1):106. https://doi.org/10.1186/s12871-018-0574-9.
8. Angus DC, Barnato AE, Linde-Zwirble WT, et al. Use of intensive care at the end of life in the United States: an epidemiologic study. Crit Care Med 2004;32(3): 638–43. https://doi.org/10.1097/01.ccm.0000114816.62331.08.
9. Schroeder K, Lorenz K. Nursing and the future of palliative care. Asia-Pac J Oncol Nurs 2018;5(1):4–8. https://doi.org/10.4103/apjon.apjon_43_17.
10. Singer AE, Goebel JR, Kim YS, et al. Populations and interventions for palliative and end-of-life care: a systematic review. J Palliat Med 2016;19(9):995–1008. https://doi.org/10.1089/jpm.2015.0367.
11. Desmedt MS, de la Kethulle YL, Deveugele MI, et al. Palliative inpatients in general hospitals: a one day observational study in Belgium. BMC Palliat Care 2011; 10:2. https://doi.org/10.1186/1472-684X-10-2.
12. Gardiner C, Gott M, Ingleton C, et al. Extent of palliative care need in the acute hospital setting: a survey of two acute hospitals in the UK. Palliat Med 2013; 27(1):76–83. https://doi.org/10.1177/0269216312447592.
13. Radbruch L, De Lima L, Knaul F, et al. Redefining palliative care—a new consensus-based definition. J Pain Symptom Manag 2020;60(4):754–64. https://doi.org/10.1016/j.jpainsymman.2020.04.027.
14. Kaasa S, Loge JH, Aapro M, et al. Title Page: Lancet Oncology Commission Title: Integration of oncology and palliative care.
15. Palliative & end-of-life care - AACN. Available at: https://www.aacn.org/clinical-resources/palliative-end-of-life. Accessed June 21, 2024.
16. Palliative care, report card. Palliative care, report card. Available at: https://reportcard.capc.org/. Accessed June 21, 2024.
17. Avati A, Jung K, Harman S, et al. Improving palliative care with deep learning. BMC Med Inf Decis Making 2018;18(S4):122. https://doi.org/10.1186/s12911-018-0677-8.
18. Sjöberg M, Edberg AK, Rasmussen BH, et al. Documentation of older people's end-of-life care in the context of specialised palliative care: a retrospective review of patient records. BMC Palliat Care 2021;20(1):91. https://doi.org/10.1186/s12904-021-00771-w.

19. Pan H, Shi W, Zhou Q, et al. Palliative care in the intensive care unit: not just end-of-life care. Intensive Care Res 2023;3(1):77–82. https://doi.org/10.1007/s44231-022-00009-0.

20. Tzenalis A, Papaemmanuel H, Kipourgos G, et al. End-of-life care in the intesive care unit and nursing roles in communicating with families. J Crit Care Med 2023; 9(2):116–21.

21. End-of-Life Nursing Education Consortium (ELNEC). (n.d.). *About ELNEC.* https://www.aacnnursing.org/elnec.

22. Rababa M, Al-Sabbah S, Hayajneh AA. Nurses' perceived barriers to and facilitators of pain assessment and management in critical care patients: a systematic review. J Pain Res 2021;14:3475–91. https://doi.org/10.2147/JPR.S332423.

23. Butkus R, Rapp K, Cooney TG, et al, Health and Public Policy Committee of the American College of Physicians. Envisioning a better U.S. Health care system for all: reducing barriers to care and addressing social determinants of health. Ann Intern Med 2020;172(2 Suppl):S50–9. https://doi.org/10.7326/M19-2410.

24. Fiscella K, Epstein RM, Griggs JJ, et al. Is physician implicit bias associated with differences in care by patient race for metastatic cancer-related pain?. In: Orueta JF, editor. PLoS One 2021;16(10):e0257794. https://doi.org/10.1371/journal.pone.0257794.

25. Rego F, Gonçalves F, Moutinho S, et al. The influence of spirituality on decision-making in palliative care outpatients: a cross-sectional study. BMC Palliat Care 2020;19(1):22. https://doi.org/10.1186/s12904-020-0525-3.

26. Brant JM, Silbermann M. Global perspectives on palliative care for cancer patients: not all countries are the same. Curr Oncol Rep 2021;23(5):60. https://doi.org/10.1007/s11912-021-01044-8.

27. Perugino F, De Angelis V, Pompili M, et al. Stigma and chronic pain. Pain Ther 2022;11(4):1085–94. https://doi.org/10.1007/s40122-022-00418-5.

28. Sinha A, Deshwal H, Vashisht R. End-of-Life evaluation and management of pain. In: *StatPearls.* Treasure Island (FL). StatPearls Publishing; 2024. Available at: http://www.ncbi.nlm.nih.gov/books/NBK568753/. Accessed June 21, 2024.

29. Wojnar-Gruszka K, Sega A, Płaszewska-Żywko L, et al. Pain assessment with the BPS and CCPOT behavioral pain scales in mechanically ventilated patients requiring analgesia and sedation. Int J Environ Res Publ Health 2022;19(17): 10894. https://doi.org/10.3390/ijerph191710894.

Orthopedic Pain Management
Tools for Practicing Critical Care Nurses

Lynn C. Parsons, PhD, RN, NEA-BC*

KEYWORDS

- Acute pain • Chronic pain • Pain by body region • Pain demographics
- Pain and discomfort in intensive care unit settings • Culture
- Resources on pain management

KEY POINTS

- The prevalence of orthopedic pain is high compared to other body regions by age, ethnicity, gender, and income per research findings.
- Nurses in intensive care units frequently manage acute and chronic orthopedic pain simultaneously.
- Many factors contribute to pain and discomfort for orthopedic patients in the intensive care unit.
- Persons from different cultures have unique pain expressions and experiences.
- There are many current Internet resources available to intensive care unit nurses and other health professionals for managing pain.

INTRODUCTION

Critical care registered nurses manage pain on a daily basis in hospital settings. Along with acute and new traumatic pain, nurses must also manage chronic pain that patients have prior to their admission to the intensive care unit (ICU).

Americans experience chronic pain in greater frequency than other health conditions, such as hypertension, diabetes, and clinical depression.[1] Research supports that multimodal, multidisciplinary treatment strategies can change the course of pain progression and improve patient care outcomes.[2]

Nurses are at the forefront of patient care in many different clinical specialty units. Nurses practicing in critical care settings often manage patients with systems failure and multiple trauma injuries that require widespread assessment and treatment skills. The purpose of this study is to share pain demographics, ethical considerations, and

Department of Nursing, Morehead State University, Center for Health, Education & Research, 316 West Second Street, 201P, Morehead, KY, USA
* Corresponding author.
E-mail address: Lynn.Parsons@mail.waldenu.edu

Crit Care Nurs Clin N Am 36 (2024) 609–617
https://doi.org/10.1016/j.cnc.2024.05.002   **ccnursing.theclinics.com**
0899-5885/24/

educational resources to provide the practicing nurse with a repertoire of information needed to knowledgeably provide patient care for patients experiencing pain.

ACUTE PAIN

No individual is alike, and their response to pain varies. Critical care nurses frequently care for persons with sudden events such as boating or motor vehicle accidents (MVAs). Patients with acute, multiple trauma require quick, comprehensive pain assessment and treatment of the underlying cause of their pain such as fracture or burns.[3]

As shared in the editorial preface, acute pain is typically associated with trauma, sepsis, surgical pain, burns and abrasions, and active childbirth. Traumatic fractures and postoperative recovery are major sources of acute pain. Pain and discomfort generally subsides once the underlying cause has been resolved and healed.

According to Comizio and Esposito,[4] medical experts agree that orthopedic pain ranks among the most painful conditions a person can go through. Medical experts agree that although the pain experienced by individuals is unique, certain health conditions are especially excruciating. These experts identify the most debilitating and painful orthopedic and orthopedic-related conditions. The reader is referred to **Table 1**.

The Cleveland Clinic[3] characterizes acute pain as a sudden discomfort triggered by a specific event or condition. This type of pain is typically associated with traumatic fractures, postoperative recovery, burns, abrasions, cuts, and active childbirth. It generally subsides once the underlying cause has been resolved and healed.

CHRONIC PAIN

In contrast, chronic pain is a persistent discomfort that may last for more than 6 months.[2] It often continues even after the initial cause has healed and is commonly linked to conditions such as arthritis, back pain, and cancer. Critical care patients frequently experience acute pain and chronic pain simultaneously. Many factors may contribute to pain in critically ill patients.

Table 1
Highest ranked orthopedic pain situations

Condition	Explanation
Trauma	MVAs, gunshot wounds, postoperative (fracture repair, joint surgery) and head and neck injuries
Trigeminal neuralgia	Caused by nerve compression and facial trauma
Postoperative pain	Fracture/multiple fracture and multiple orthopedic trauma associated with surgical repair
Back injuries	Disk fracture and disk herniation associate with traumatic events
Major joint osteoarthritis	Associated with chronicity—loss of the cartilage that cushions the bone and joints
Complex regional pain syndrome	Excruciating pain associated with trauma to peripheral nerves. Often seen in arm and leg injuries caused by fracture, sprain, postoperative and immobility associated with the same
Bone cancer	From either primary cancer (most prevalent sites are breast, prostate, kidney, and lung) or bone metastasis

Adapted from Comizio, C. & Esposito, L. (2024). Ranking the most painful medical conditions. UN News & World Report-Health. Available at: https://health.usnews.com/health-care/patient-advice/slideshows/ranking-the-most-painful-medical-conditions?onepage.

Approximately 51.6 million Americans experience chronic pain every day.[5] Each patient's pain experience is unique to them. Nurses practicing in critical care settings must manage a critical care event while simultaneously be able to intervene with a critical pain event that brought a patient to an ICU.

In 2019, the National Center for Health Statistics and National Health Interview Survey[6] reported findings for adults aged over 18 years and cited the body region for pain. Orthopedic pain is prevalent as the pain cause. **Fig. 1** portrays adult pain reports based upon household interviews of a sample of the civilian noninstitutionalized population in a 3 month period.

Findings from the National Center for Health Statistics and National Health Interview Survey[6] also supported that certain demographic factors contributed to pain in lower limbs (**Fig. 2**) and upper limbs (**Fig. 3**). Different cultures have different responses to pain, and nurses need to be cognizant on cultural influences related to pain and the patient's response to pain from different backgrounds.

Culture influences the patient's pain experience and how health professional manage pain.[7] Culture influences perception, expression, and how health professionals treat patient pain. A person's cultural background impacts a person's reaction and behavioral response based upon past life experiences, personal beliefs, and individual characteristics. For example, an Asian or Hispanic person experiencing significant pain may maintain a stoic or neutral demeanor despite being in significant pain. Care providers must be aware of how different cultural groups respond to pain, be aware of their own personal bias toward pain, and treat patients with dignity.

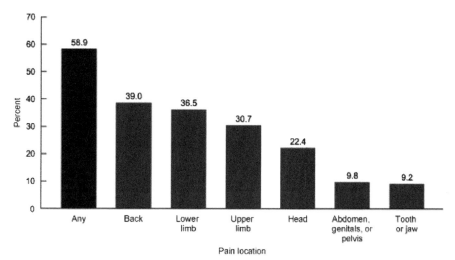

Fig. 1. Percentage of adults aged 18 years and over with any pain and pain by body region in the past 3 months: United States, 2019. *Notes:* Any pain is based on responses of "some days," "most days," or "every day" to a question asking how often the respondent had pain in the past 3 months. Pain at specific locations is based on responses of "a little," "a lot," or "somewhere between a little and a lot" to a question asking how much pain they had at these locations: (1) back; (2) hips, knees, and feet; (3) hands, arms, and shoulders; (4) headache or migraine; (5) abdomen, genitals, and pelvis; and (6) tooth and jaw. Respondents could indicate pain at more than one location. Estimates are based on household interviews of a sample of the civilian noninstitutionalized population. (National Center for Health Statistics, National Health Interview Survey, 2019.)

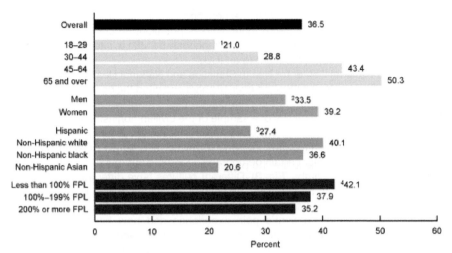

Fig. 2. Percentage of adults aged 18 years and over with pain in the hips, knees, and feet (lower limbs) in the past 3 months, by age, sex, race and Hispanic origin, and family income as a percentage of the federal poverty level: United States, 2019. *Notes*: Lower limb pain is based on responses of "a little," "a lot," or "somewhere between a little and a lot" to a question asking about how much pain they had in their hips, knees, and feet. Estimates are based on household interviews of a sample of the civilian noninstitutionalized population. FPL, federal poverty level. (National Center for Health Statistics, National Health Interview Survey, 2019.)

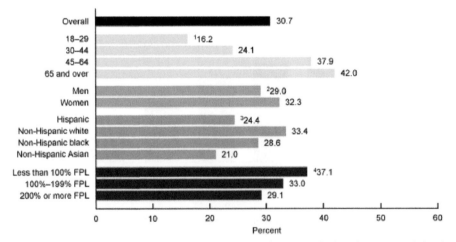

Fig. 3. Percentage of adults aged 18 years and over with pain in the hands, arms, and shoulders (upper limbs) in the past 3 months, by age, sex, race and Hispanic origin, and family income as a percentage of the federal poverty level: United States, 2019. *Notes*: Upper limb pain is based on responses of "a little," "a lot," or "somewhere between a little and a lot" to a question asking how much pain they had in their hands, arms, and shoulders. Estimates are based on household interviews of a sample of the civilian noninstitutionalized population. FPL, federal poverty level. (National Center for Health Statistics, National Health Interview Survey, 2019.)

CONTRIBUTING FACTORS FOR PATIENT PAIN IN THE INTENSIVE CARE UNIT

Critical care nurses must be aware of many dynamics inherent to patients newly admitted to the ICU that impact patients' pain experience. The factors can have a significant effect on the patient's experience, especially when occurring in combination. An example may include the patient experiencing acute orthopedic pain and grieving over loss of life of a family member that died due to injuries received in an MVA. The reader is referred to **Box 1** for factors that contribute to pain and discomfort for critically ill or injured persons.

ETHICAL RESPONSIBILITIES

Nurses have an ethical responsibility to deliver principled, individualized patient care regardless of any patient circumstance. The American Nurses Association (ANA) has a position statement that provides ethical guidance for fulfilling their obligation to provide the best care possible for persons experiencing pain.[8,9]

Major points within the ANA position statement for ethical guidance include

Box 1	
Aspects contributing to patient pain and discomfort in intensive care unit settings	
Biological	1. Symptoms of acute pain associated with fractures, burns, abrasions, and degloving injuries
	2. Wounds and abrasions: road rash associated to scrape injuries and gravel in skin post-MVA, posttrauma, and postoperative
	3. Insomnia/sleep insufficiency
	4. Temperature fluctuations often associated with interrupted skin integrity, methicillin-resistant *Staphylococcus aureus* infection that occurs around implanted hardware (often associated with metal hardware)
	5. Immobility due to traction, wound drainage tubes, intravenous or central line placement, electrocardiogram (EKG) monitors, and so forth
Psychosocial	1. Grieving
	2. Insufficient rest/sleep/relaxation
	3. Anxiety associated with loss of earnings, family role, pain reaction(s), fear of disfigurement, and physical disability
	4. Fear of dying, family member dying if in a multiperson MVA
	5. Separation from friends, family, coworkers, and church family
	6. Lack of pleasurable outlets, boredom
	7. Fearful of pain, worried about current and future pain management
ICU atmosphere	1. Unfamiliar noises, public address systems, equipment sounds, staff member communications, and voices of visitors in other rooms
	2. Ultraviolet lighting
	3. Equipment lights
	4. Being woke up for ICU routines, for example, emptying wound vacuum-assisted closure, hanging intravenous fluids, and turning/repositioning
	5. Priorities that interfere with pain management include airway management, hemorrhagic events, abnormal EKG, and unstable vital signs

Table 2
Online resources for pain management

Association	Web Site	Resource Description
American Society for Pain Management in Nursing	http://www.aspmn.org/	Professional nurses dedicated to promoting and providing optimal care of individuals with pain, including its aftermath
American Academy of Pain Medicine	https://painmed.org/american-pain-society/	Advances multidisciplinary pain care, technology, education, and advocacy
American Chronic Pain Association	www.theacpa.org	Education and advocacy support for persons with chronic pain conditions
American Pain Foundation	www.painfoundation.com	Information for the general public/patients and their families, health care professionals, media, legislators, and caregivers
City of Hope Pain/Palliative Care Resource Center	https://prc.coh.org	Resources to assist with improving pain management and end-of-life care; a source for patient education materials, quality management tools, and research instruments
National Guideline Clearinghouse	https://www.ahrq.gov/gam/index.html	Resources for evidence-based clinical practice guidelines for pain sponsored n = by the Agency for Healthcare Research and Quality (AHRQ)
Center to Advance Palliative Care	www.capc.org	Contains national data for prevalence of palliative care platforms, consumer information, and quality management resources

- Nurses are ethically responsible to assess and relieve pain and determine causes of pain.
- The scientific problem-solving model, "The Nursing Process," should guide nursing practice interventions.
- Nurses should provide individualized patient care.
- Multimodal and interdisciplinary approaches are needed to achieve pain control and pain relief.
- Pain-management practices should be guided by current evidenced-based literature.
- Nurse must be advocates and engage legislators to secure access to effective policies.
- Nurse leadership is requisite in society to address addiction and specifically the opioid crisis.

Nurses must acknowledge patients' pain and their description of pain, assess the source of pain, and monitor pain at frequent intervals. They shoulder the responsibility of managing pain in critical care settings.[10] The following are key components to assess the patient for biological, psychological, and emotional signs of patient pain and discomfort.

- Groaning, crying, and verbalizations, for example, "No!"
- Decreased movement in bed
- Facial and body images, for example, tightened face, crying, and clenched fists
- Sudden behavior changes
- Increasing irritability
- Protecting a body part, for example, protecting a sore limb

RESOURCES FOR CRITICAL CARE NURSES RELEVANT TO PAIN MANAGEMENT

Maintaining currency in critical care nursing and knowing new and innovative pain-management strategies is a major responsibility for the practicing nurse. Involvement in professional nursing organizations, reading current evidence-based literature and accessing online information sources are essential to safe and competent critical care nursing practice.

There are also several Internet resources that should be accessed to maintain current information available in managing pain. These resources include information for the lay public, caregivers, patients and their family members, health care professionals, the media, and our elected officials. Furthermore, these resources will also share information about conferences specific to pain management, new educational resources, quality improvement mechanisms, current pain practice standards, guidelines, and position statements that address pain-management assessment and treatment strategies.

The reader is referred to **Table 2** to view Internet resources that address pain management, links to access information specific to the resource, and a brief description of information contained in individual Web sites.

SUMMARY

Critical care nurses need a strong skill set to best manage traumatic, acute, and chronic orthopedic pain. They must be able to manage all pain types simultaneously. There are many facets that contribute to patient pain, and astute critical nurses manage these factors to achieve optimal patient outcomes. Awareness of patient demographics, which includes cultural knowledge and awareness, is important for nurses to maintain in their skill repertoire when managing orthopedic pain in ICUs. Nurses must act ethically in delivering care to persons in pain to minimize pain and promote optimal care outcomes. The ANA position statement guides nurses in their ethical responsibilities in managing pain and suffering. Finally, nurses must constantly update their knowledge and skills to manage critically injured orthopedic patients. The Internet is a rich resource for current, cutting-edge, evidenced-based research findings that support optimal care delivery.

CLINICS CARE POINTS

- Critical care nurses must treat traumatic, acute, and chronic pain in ICU settings.
- Patient's response and expression to pain is individualized and is impacted by cultural differences.
- Critical care nurses must be aware of all factors that contribute to pain and mitigate the impact of these issues.
- The ANA position statement for managing pain should be used as a guide for critical care nurses.
- Current resource acquisition is required to deliver current, competent, intensive care to orthopedic patients in pain.

DISCLOSURE

The author reports no commercial or financial conflicts of interest. There was no funding from any source for this publication.

REFERENCES

1. U.S. Department of Health and Human Services. NIH study finds high rates of persistent chronic pain among U.S. adults. Washngton, DC: National Institute of Health; 2023.
2. Nahin RL, Feinberg T, Kapos FP, et al. Estimated rates of incident and persistent chronic pain among US adults, 2019-2020. JAMA Netw Open 2023. https://doi.org/10.1001/jamanetworkopen.2023.13563 (link is external).
3. Cleveland Clinic (December 8. Acute vs. Chronic pain. 2020. Available at: https://my.clevelandclinic.org/health/articles/12051-acute-vs-chronic-pain. [Accessed 4 January 2024].
4. Comizio C, Esposito L. Ranking the most painful medical conditions. UN News & World Report-Health 2024. Available at: https://health.usnews.com/health-care/patient-advice/slideshows/ranking-the-most-painful-medical-conditions?one page.
5. US Pain Foundation. The impact of pain in America. 2023. Available at: https://uspainfoundation.org/news/the-impact-of-pain-in-america/.
6. National Center for Health Statistics. National health interview Survey. 2019. Available at: https://www.cdc.gov/nchs/nhis/index.htm.
7. Rogger R, Bello C, Romero CS, et al. Cultural framing and the impact on acute pain and pain services. Curr Pain Headache Rep 2023;27:429–36.
8. Stokes J. ANA position statement: the ethical responsibility to manage pain and the suffering it causes. Onl Jrnl of Issues in Nsg. Available at: https://www.nursingworld.

org/practice-policy/nursing-excellence/official-position-statements/id/the-ethical-responsibility-to-manage-pain-and-the-suffering-it-causes/.

9. American Nurses Association. Code of ethics for nurses. Silver Springs, MD: American Nurses Publishing; 2015.
10. Morton P, Thurman P. Critical care nursing: a holistic approach. 12th edition. Alphen aan den Rijn, the Netherlands: Wolters Kluwer; 2024.

UNITED STATES POSTAL SERVICE® Statement of Ownership, Management, and Circulation
(All Periodicals Publications Except Requester Publications)

1. Publication Title CRITICAL CARE NURSING CLINICS OF NORTH AMERICA	**2. Publication Number** 006 – 273	**3. Filing Date** 9/18/24
4. Issue Frequency MAR, JUN SEP, DEC	**5. Number of Issues Published Annually** 4	**6. Annual Subscription Price** $166.00

7. Complete Mailing Address of Known Office of Publication (Not printer) (Street, city, county, state, and ZIP+4®)
ELSEVIER INC.
230 Park Avenue, Suite 800
New York, NY 10169

Contact Person: Malathi Samayan
Telephone (Include area code): 91-44-4299-4507

8. Complete Mailing Address of Headquarters or General Business Office of Publisher (Not printer)
ELSEVIER INC.
230 Park Avenue, Suite 800
New York, NY 10169

9. Full Names and Complete Mailing Addresses of Publisher, Editor, and Managing Editor (Do not leave blank)

Publisher (Name and complete mailing address)
DOLORES MELONI, ELSEVIER INC.
1600 JOHN F KENNEDY BLVD. SUITE 1600
PHILADELPHIA, PA 19103-2899

Editor (Name and complete mailing address)
KERRY HOLLAND, ELSEVIER INC.
1600 JOHN F KENNEDY BLVD. SUITE 1600
PHILADELPHIA, PA 19103-2899

Managing Editor (Name and complete mailing address)
PATRICK MANLEY, ELSEVIER INC.
1600 JOHN F KENNEDY BLVD. SUITE 1600
PHILADELPHIA, PA 19103-2899

10. Owner (Do not leave blank. If the publication is owned by a corporation, give the name and address of the corporation immediately followed by the names and addresses of all stockholders owning or holding 1 percent or more of the total amount of stock. If not owned by a corporation, give the names and addresses of the individual owners. If owned by a partnership or other unincorporated firm, give its name and address as well as those of each individual owner. If the publication is published by a nonprofit organization, give its name and address.)

Full Name	Complete Mailing Address
WHOLLY OWNED SUBSIDIARY OF REED/ELSEVIER, US HOLDINGS	1600 JOHN F KENNEDY BLVD. SUITE 1600 PHILADELPHIA, PA 19103-2899

11. Known Bondholders, Mortgagees, and Other Security Holders Owning or Holding 1 Percent or More of Total Amount of Bonds, Mortgages, or Other Securities. If none, check box ▶ ☐ None

Full Name	Complete Mailing Address
N/A	

12. Tax Status (For completion by nonprofit organizations authorized to mail at nonprofit rates) (Check one)
The purpose, function, and nonprofit status of this organization and the exempt status for federal income tax purposes:
☒ Has Not Changed During Preceding 12 Months
☐ Has Changed During Preceding 12 Months (Publisher must submit explanation of change with this statement)

PS Form **3526**, July 2014 [Page 1 of 4 (see instructions page 4)] PSN: 7530-01-000-9931   PRIVACY NOTICE: See our privacy policy on www.usps.com.

13. Publication Title	14. Issue Date for Circulation Data below
CRITICAL CARE NURSING CLINICS OF NORTH AMERICA	JUNE 2024

15. Extent and Nature of Circulation		Average No. Copies Each Issue During Preceding 12 Months	No. Copies of Single Issue Published Nearest to Filing Date
a. Total Number of Copies (Net press run)		84	70
b. Paid Circulation (By Mail and Outside the Mail)	(1) Mailed Outside-County Paid Subscriptions Stated on PS Form 3541 (Include paid distribution above nominal rate, advertiser's proof copies, and exchange copies)	53	38
	(2) Mailed In-County Paid Subscriptions Stated on PS Form 3541 (Include paid distribution above nominal rate, advertiser's proof copies, and exchange copies)	0	0
	(3) Paid Distribution Outside the Mails Including Sales Through Dealers and Carriers, Street Vendors, Counter Sales, and Other Paid Distribution Outside USPS®	18	18
	(4) Paid Distribution by Other Classes of Mail Through the USPS (e.g. First-Class Mail®)	6	6
c. Total Paid Distribution [Sum of 15b (1), (2), (3), and (4)]	▶	77	62
d. Free or Nominal Rate Distribution (By Mail and Outside the Mail)	(1) Free or Nominal Rate Outside-County Copies included on PS Form 3541	7	7
	(2) Free or Nominal Rate In-County Copies Included on PS Form 3541	0	0
	(3) Free or Nominal Rate Copies Mailed at Other Classes Through the USPS (e.g. First-Class Mail)	0	0
	(4) Free or Nominal Rate Distribution Outside the Mail (Carriers or other means)	1	1
e. Total Free or Nominal Rate Distribution (Sum of 15d (1), (2), (3) and (4))	▶	8	8
f. Total Distribution (Sum of 15c and 15e)	▶	84	70
g. Copies not Distributed (See Instructions to Publishers #4 (page #3))	▶	0	0
h. Total (Sum of 15f and g)	▶	84	70
i. Percent Paid (15c divided by 15f times 100)		91.07%	88.57%

* If you are claiming electronic copies, go to line 16 on page 3. If you are not claiming electronic copies, skip to line 17 on page 3.

PS Form **3526**, July 2014 (Page 2 of 4)

16. Electronic Copy Circulation		Average No. Copies Each Issue During Preceding 12 Months	No. Copies of Single Issue Published Nearest to Filing Date
a. Paid Electronic Copies	▶		
b. Total Paid Print Copies (Line 15c) + Paid Electronic Copies (Line 16a)	▶		
c. Total Print Distribution (Line 15f) + Paid Electronic Copies (Line 16a)	▶		
d. Percent Paid (Both Print & Electronic Copies) (16b divided by 16c × 100)	▶		

☒ I certify that 50% of all my distributed copies (electronic and print) are paid above a nominal price.

17. Publication of Statement of Ownership
☒ If the publication is a general publication, publication of this statement is required. Will be printed in the DECEMBER 2024 issue of this publication.
☐ Publication not required.

18. Signature and Title of Editor, Publisher, Business Manager or Owner

Malathi Samayan - Distribution Controller

Malathi Samayan   Date 9/18/24

I certify that all information furnished on this form is true and complete. I understand that anyone who furnishes false or misleading information on this form or who omits material or information requested on the form may be subject to criminal sanctions (including fines and imprisonment) and/or civil sanctions (including civil penalties).

PS Form **3526**, July 2014 (Page 3 of 4)   PRIVACY NOTICE: See our privacy policy on www.usps.com

Moving?

Make sure your subscription moves with you!

To notify us of your new address, find your **Clinics Account Number** (located on your mailing label above your name), and contact customer service at:

Email: journalscustomerservice-usa@elsevier.com

800-654-2452 (subscribers in the U.S. & Canada)
314-447-8871 (subscribers outside of the U.S. & Canada)

Fax number: 314-447-8029

Elsevier Health Sciences Division
Subscription Customer Service
3251 Riverport Lane
Maryland Heights, MO 63043

*To ensure uninterrupted delivery of your subscription, please notify us at least 4 weeks in advance of move.

Printed and bound by CPI Group (UK) Ltd, Croydon, CR0 4YY

08/05/2025

01864751-0008